Clinical Pathways
for Collaborative
Practice

Clinical Pathways
for Collaborative
Practice

DONNA D. IGNATAVICIUS, MS, RNC

Instructor, MacQueen Gibbs Willis School of Nursing
Consultant, DI Associates
Easton, Maryland

KATHY A. HAUSMAN, MS, RNC, CNRN

Director of Education Services
Harbor Hospital Center
Baltimore, Maryland

W.B. SAUNDERS COMPANY

A Division of Harcourt Brace & Company

Philadelphia   London   Toronto   Montreal   Sydney   Tokyo

W.B. SAUNDERS COMPANY

A Division of Harcourt Brace & Company

The Curtis Center
Independence Square West
Philadelphia, Pennsylvania 19106

Library of Congress Cataloging-in-Publication Data

Ignatavicius, Donna D.
    Clinical pathways for collaborative practice / Donna D.
Ignatavicius, Kathy A. Hausman, — 1st ed.
      p.   cm.
   ISBN 0-7216-4741-3
   1. Medical protocols. 2. Health care teams. 3. Hospitals—Case
management services.   I. Hausman, Kathy A.   II. Title.
   [DNLM: 1. Patient Care Team. 2. Diagnosis. 3. Patient Care
Planning. 4. Managed Care Programs.   W 84.8 I24c 1995]
RC64.I36 1995
362.1'068—dc20
DNLM/DLC
                           95-3461

Last digit is the print number: 9   8   7   6   5   4   3   2   1

To Stephanie, for having an enormous amount of patience while I spent many hours working on this project—I love you very much!

DDI

To Wayne, for bringing me snacks when I was trying to meet my deadlines; and to the staff at Harbor Hospital Center who provided my inspiration for this book.

KAH

Reviewers

Shannon McDowell Bailey, MS, RN, HCRM
Affiliated Risk Control Administrators
Tampa, Florida

Patricia Marie Barnes, BSN, RN, ONC
William Beaumont Hospital
Royal Oak, Michigan

Marilyn A. Cummings, MS, RN
Rush Presbyterian St. Luke's Medical Center
Chicago, Illinois

Beverly Cunningham, MS, RN
Case Management Consultants
Oologah, Oklahoma

Eileen Connor Finnegan, BSN, RN, CCRN
American Association of Critical-Care Nurses
Aliso Viejo, California
Our Lady of Lourdes Medical Center
Camden, New Jersey

Marilyn A. Folcik, MPH, RN, ONC
Hartford Hospital
Hartford, Connecticut

Anna Gawlinski, DNSc, RN, CS, CCRN
University of California Medical Center
Los Angeles, California

Karen Bigos Graybeal, MS, RN
Good Samaritan Hospital
Puyallup, Washington

Louise Grondin, MS, RN
University of Michigan Hospitals
Ann Arbor, Michigan

Margaret Hickey, MS, RN
Rush Presbyterian St. Luke's Medical Center
Chicago, Illinois

Laurel D. Kersten, PhD, RN
University of Colorado Health Sciences Center
Denver, Colorado

Deanna Kruckenberg, RN, OCN
Oncology Nursing Society
Washington Nurses Society
Tacoma, Washington

Cynthia D. Marion, BSC, RN, OCN
Good Samaritan Community Health Care
Puyallup, Washington

M. Erin McKenna, BScN, RN
The Toronto Hospital
Toronto, Ontario
Canada

Barbara J. Riegel, DNSc, RN, CS, FAAN
Clinical Researcher
Sharp Health Care
San Diego, California

Mary F. Rodts, MS, RN, ONC
Assistant Professor
Rush University
Chicago, Illinois

Susan Moeller Schneider, MS, RN, CS, OCN
Doctoral Student
Frances Payne Bolton School of Nursing
Case Western Reserve University
Cleveland, Ohio

Penny Lynn Tice, MSN, RN, CS, CCRN
Baptist Memorial Hospital
University of Tennessee
Memphis, Tennessee

Pamela Becker Weilitz, MSN(R), RN
Barnes Hospital
St. Louis University School of Nursing
University of Missouri, Kansas City
St. Louis Graduate Nursing Program Faculty
St. Louis, Missouri

Judy E. White, MA, MSN, RN
Rockland Community College
Suffern, New York

Preface

Over the past 4 years, we have had a keen interest in clinical pathways. Donna's experience with pathways as a clinical instructor and Kathy's experience as a facilitator for pathway development have enabled us to write a book that we feel will be useful to clinicians, administrators, students, and educators.

Clinicians, including case managers and staff nurses, and administrators of health care agencies will find that Chapters 1 through 5 walk them through the process of clinical pathway development, implementation, evaluation, and revision. Although the generic pathways in Parts II and III are directed primarily towards acute care, samples in Chapter 4 illustrate how pathways are being used in alternate care settings.

We think that students and educators will also benefit from this book. Students rarely have the opportunity to follow a patient through a complete episode of care. Clinical pathways display the entire treatment plan and show students where their individual care "fits in" as part of the interdisciplinary plan of care.

Educators can use pathways as teaching tools, both in the classroom and clinical settings. Once students are grounded in the nursing process and understand their practice role, they can then conceptualize patient care on a broader scale—in collaboration with their health care colleagues.

The book is divided into three major parts. Part I encompasses five chapters that discuss the concept of clinical pathways. Chapter 1 introduces the reader to managed care, case management, and clinical pathways and explains the relationship between and among these elements. Chapter 2 describes the pathway development process in detail, offering practical suggestions and ways to avoid pitfalls. Chapter 3 discusses variance monitoring and analysis. Chapter 4 presents various ways in which pathways are being used around the United States, and Chapter 5 outlines the format for the clinical pathways used in this book.

Parts II and III contain sample clinical pathways organized by body system. Part II has pathways for common diagnoses seen in the acute medical-surgical setting. Part III has pathways for common diagnoses seen in the critical care setting.

Patient versions of six pathways in English and five in Spanish are located in the Appendices. These pathways can be copied and used as you need. We also included a list of abbreviations that are used in the generic pathways in Parts II and III and the most recently approved NANDA nursing diagnosis list.

We hope that you enjoy this book and find it helpful as you develop and implement clinical pathways in your setting.

Donna D. Ignatavicius
Kathy A. Hausman

Acknowledgments

We wish to thank the following individuals for their help and expertise.

From the Harbor Hospital Center, Baltimore, MD—Jan Zeller, Nursing Case Manager; Elizabeth Oakley, Coder II, Medical Records; Jane Nykiel, Quality Management Specialist; Dr. Calvin Fuhrman, Chief, Division of Pulmonology; Sharon Powers, Nursing Administration Secretary; and the Wound Care Team.

From W.B. Saunders—Barbara Nelson Cullen, Nursing Editor; Francine Rosenthal, Editorial Assistant; Joan Sinclair, Production Manager.

From Cracom Corporation—Joy Moore, Production Editor.

Finally, Esperanza Villanueva Joyce, EdD, RN, for the Spanish translation and review of the terminology.

Contents

Part III
Clinical Pathways for Critical Care Patients

Unit IX

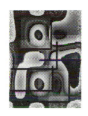

Part I

Introduction to Clinical Pathways

Introduction to Case Management and Clinical Pathways

The delivery of health care in the United States is rapidly changing. The 1990s have seen decreased lengths of hospital stays; sicker patients admitted to hospitals; increased use of ambulatory services, including same-day surgery; and sicker patients in alternate care settings such as home health and long-term care. Health care agencies, health insurers, and employers continue to seek alternative ways to provide high-quality care in a cost-effective manner.

Managed care, case management, and clinical pathways are "hot" trends in patient care management in the 1990s. Their purpose is to promote quality patient care while controlling costs. Everyone has a different view, however, about what these trends are, how they should be used, and how to implement them in a health care setting. Although there are no universal definitions, each trend can be described generically.

MANAGED CARE

Health insurance companies have looked at the cost of patient care and recognized the need for a better health care delivery system—managed care. Managed care includes a collection of strategies such as prepayment arrangements and preadmission authorizations used by purchasers of health care to control costs. In a managed care system a case manager acts as a gatekeeper and follows a patient through the system. The patient's primary physician typically authorizes when use of a specialist or other health service is necessary.

Managed care encompasses a wide variety of organizational structures such as health maintenance organizations (HMOs) and preferred provider organizations (PPOs) (Hicks, Stallmeyer, and Coleman, 1992). Discussion of insurance-based managed care is beyond the scope of this book, but several references can be found in the bibliography at the end of Part I.

CASE MANAGEMENT

Description of Case Management

Although some references imply that case management is a branch of, type of, or the same as managed care, this book distinguishes the two concepts to avoid

3

confusion for the reader. In contrast to insurance-based managed care, case management is a *practice model* that uses a systematic approach to identify specific patients and to manage patient care to ensure optimum outcomes.

Within the past decade, case management has been introduced into the inpatient setting as a model for restructuring patient care delivery to improve cost and quality outcomes. Until the early 1980s, health care delivery was fragmented, which resulted in high costs, prolonged lengths of stays in hospitals, and unnecessary use of health care resources. Physicians varied their practice according to their specific experiences and professional styles. Discharge planning often did not begin until the day of discharge from the hospital, resulting in lack of patient teaching and essential planning to ensure continuity of care.

Because hospitals in the United States were reimbursed for health care on a dollar-for-dollar basis by third-party payors (e.g., private health insurers, Medicare), there was little incentive for hospitals to change their way of providing care. In 1982, however, the introduction of prospective payment and competitive bidding stimulated an interest in reducing hospital costs while optimizing patient care outcomes.

Case management is an alternative to fragmented, high-cost care. Patient care services provided by the interdisciplinary team are coordinated by a case manager or case coordinator. Various health care disciplines are scrambling to claim ownership of case management (Williams, 1992).

Nurses have long recognized the need for case management. In some settings they have developed nursing case management (NCM) as a system for implementing the nursing process in collaboration with other health team members. In NCM the nurse's goal is to meet the multiple needs of patients in multiple health care settings with multiple caregivers. In other words, NCM is based on the premise that client care must be carefully coordinated across a continuum of care settings (Bower, 1992).

Early Models of Case Management

The earliest models for NCM were developed in the mid-1980s (Table 1–1). The first published model was developed in 1985 at the New England Medical Center in Boston, Massachusetts, where Karen Zander and Kathy Bower pioneered "second-generation primary nursing." In this unit-based clinical model the direct care provider is the primary (professional) nurse case manager. Collaborative group practice with physicians and other health care professionals is "episode based," or as needed for patient care.

In 1986 Carondelet St. Mary's Hospital and Health Center in Tucson, Arizona, created an NCM model that expands beyond the walls of the hospital into

TABLE 1–1 **Early Models for Nursing Case Management**

New England Medical Center	Carondelet St. Mary's Hospital and Health Center
Unit-based model	Integrated system of nursing care that spans the health care continuum; may be unit or episode based
Staff (primary) nurse driven	Nursing group practice, including clinical specialists and educators
Hospital oriented	Inside and outside the walls of the hospital; community health centers
Collaborative group practice (nurses and physicians)	Health promotion is a primary feature, with focus on transcultural and spiritual health

community health centers. This model reflects health promotion with a focus on transcultural and spiritual care. Carondelet's model is particularly appropriate for its large community population of Hispanic and Native Americans.

Since the work of these two early nursing case management developers, many variations of case management have been engineered. Some models are not *nursing* case management. Instead, they are referred to as *care management, collaborative management, managed care,* or *collaborative care* to illustrate the collaborative, interdisciplinary nature of patient care.

Some case management models are clinically oriented; other models, such as St. Peter's Medical Center Care Management Model in New Brunswick, New Jersey, are business oriented. A business-oriented model focuses on selected groups of patients to decrease costs by reducing hospital lengths of stay. Detailed information about various models of case management can be found in *Hospital Case Management* (American Health Consultants) newsletters and in the references supplied in the bibliography of Part I.

Benefits of Case Management

Nearly all hospitals that have published case management models have shown a decrease in length of stay (LOS) and significant cost savings. For example, at Hennepin County Medical Center in Minneapolis, Minnesota, the LOS in the intensive care unit for major bowel procedures decreased from 14 days (before case management) to 6 days (after case management). The readmission rate also dropped from 26% to 6% (Bower, 1992).

In addition to cost savings, customer (patient) satisfaction and staff satisfaction have improved in many settings, according to anecdotal accounts. Third-party payors, especially health insurance companies, have also encouraged the use of case management by offering discounts or other incentives to hospitals who use it. Some companies have employed physicians and other health care professionals to foster the development of case management systems in hospital settings.

The Joint Commission on the Accreditation of Healthcare Organizations (JCAHO) has also been supportive of case management as a way of delivering care. JCAHO guidelines for 1995 require an interdisciplinary, collaborative approach to patient care. Case management provides for collaboration among all members of the health care team.

Other advantages of case management reported in the literature include improved quality of care, improved communication among health team members, and decreased staff absenteeism and turnover (Cohen, 1991).

Dilemmas Associated With Case Management

Although the concept of case management appears to be the ideal practice model for health care, several areas of concern and controversy remain. First, which model is the best for the agency? Does the use of a nursing case management model reflect interdisciplinary patient care?

Second, who should the case manager be? Many hospitals use nurses, either baccalaureate or masters prepared, as case managers. Lourdes Hospital in Binghamton, New York, employs 10 masters-prepared clinical nurse specialists as case managers. The caseload is 16 to 36 patients per case manager. The project director asserts that physicians find these nurses very credible because they are clinical experts with a broad knowledge base (*Hospital Case Management,* September 1993).

Not everyone agrees that nurses are the only health care professionals who qualify as case managers, although most agencies use nurses in this capacity.

```
                     HARBOR HOSPITAL CENTER


                     POSITION DESCRIPTION

Position Number   589            TITLE   Clinical Specialist I
                                         NURSING CASE MANAGER

Exempt Status    Exempt          Division  Nursing
Hours _____   Cost Center _____
```

I. Primary Function

The Nursing Case Manager (NCM) is responsible for the daily planning, coordination, and monitoring of care with the nursing staff and other health care professionals caring for the patient.

Responsible for developing care for the caseload assigned. Accountable for assuring effective use of available resources, maintaining established standards of care and meeting outcomes within an appropriate length of stay. Ensures that variations based on patients' individual needs are justified and well documented.

II. Minimum Qualifications

Education: Graduate of an accredited school of nursing. BSN preferred; MSN preferred.

Certification: Current MD RN license. Certification in clinical specialty appropriate to the units assigned patient population. (Must be obtained within 2 years of appointment.)

Experience: Three to 5 years experience in a clinical specialty appropriate to the unit's assigned patient population. Experience in clinical instruction

III. Scope of Practice

The nursing case manager (NCM) will establish personal networks to collaborate with other departments to achieve the defined patient outcomes that the case management team seeks in meeting the needs of our patients. The NCM will work with physicians and other members of the health care team in developing and negotiating protocols that reconcile criteria set from both diagnostic and reimbursement perspectives.

IV. Duties

A. Clinical   70%

1. Admits patients arriving on assigned shift, assessing their nursing needs.

2. Contacts physician(s) to begin sharing assessments, goals, and plans for the patient's episode of illness.

3. Knows the anticipated DRG, length of stay, and transfer or discharge date.

FIGURE 1–1 Sample job description for a nurse case manager. (Courtesy of Harbor Hospital Center, Baltimore, Maryland.)

4. Familiarizes self with assigned patient's medical history and keeps track of the major sequence of events in current hospitalization.

5. Collaborates daily with the RN or LPN direct care givers in pursuing the nursing process (including teaching rounds as indicated) for assigned patients and assists in direct care when necessary.

6. Assumes responsibility for ongoing assessment of patient care needs through frequent patient rounds and communication with clinical leader, clinical specialist, direct nursing caregivers, physicians, and other members of the health care team.

7. Reviews the care plan/clinical pathway with the direct care givers. Evaluates outcomes and initiates any modification in plans necessitated by the patient's condition and with physician approval as appropriate.

8. Identifies specific parameters to be monitored to prevent complications. Initiates appropriate nursing orders to this end.

9. Monitors charts and nursing documentation for fulfillment of nursing standards and consistency in reporting.

10. Evaluates care according to practice standards, policies, and expected patient outcomes.

11. Accurately assesses problems and goal identification, which includes the patient's and family's perceptions and concerns.

12. Selects initial care plan and critical pathway, if established, and coordinates discharge plans with appropriate departments.

13. Compares the standard case management plan against the patient's individual needs in such areas as social and economic data, family resources, functional abilities, knowledge needs, potential risk factors and complications, and special issues.

14. Reviews and revises the individual critical pathway with the physician(s) within 24 hours of admission.

15. Contacts other key members of the patient's team (e.g., social worker, dietician, physical therapist).

16. Negotiates and sequences care contribution with other hospital services (e.g., radiology, respiratory therapy, patient transport) for logical order and timely response.

17. Accompanies and assists physicians on rounds. Keeps them informed about current patient status. Consults with them on patient progress toward expected outcomes.

FIGURE 1–1 *Continued*

Continued on following page.

18. Discusses with the patient and family the critical pathway, sequence of events, patient progress, and outcomes that they can reasonably expect.

19. Documents the achievement of intermediate goals and clinical outcomes as they occur.

20. Evaluates and collaborates with all members of the health care team to document patient status and variances, working toward achievement of patient goals and expected outcomes.

21. Requests consultation and feedback before a crisis occurs.

22. Plans, participates in, and follows through with health care team meetings, as needed.

23. Communicates daily with family on patient status, progress toward expected outcomes, satisfaction with services, and postdischarge planning.

24. Coordinates patient and family education in preparation for discharge.

25. Telephones patient or family 24-48 hours after discharge to ascertain status and resolve any problems within nursing scope of responsibility.

26. Completes the necessary forms in the event of a patient transfer to another health care facility and provides follow-up with phone calls to sustain continuity of care.

27. Identifies and/or coordinates the resources that the patient may need upon discharge.

28. Ensures that discharge teaching is completed and documented.

29. Attends and presents cases at discharge planning meetings.

30. Assures that the plan of care has been developed and team members are meeting the needs of the patients as they progress through the critical pathway.

31. Performs other related duties as required.

B. Quality Assurance, Research and Education   20%

   1. Carries out identified quality assurance and quality improvement initiatives.

   2. Incorporates current nursing research findings into implementation of care per hospital policies and procedures.

   3. Participates in department-wide educational programs and in-services.

FIGURE 1–1 *Continued*

4. Enhances understanding of the nurse case management process through availability and interactions with patients, families, and all members of the health care team.

C. Professional and Personal Development   10%

    1. Pursues professional education to maintain current clinical competence in a chosen field of concentration.

    2. Completes all of the required yearly educational updates.

    3. Identifies own areas of strength and opportunities for growth.

    4. Demonstrates behaviors consistent with Harbor Hospital Center philosophy and the Family Touch Standards of Conduct.

    5. Engenders confidence of patients, staff, and community through appearance and behavior, and by serving as a positive role model.

V. Supervision Received

Direct supervision is provided by the Director of Nursing of the assigned area.

VI. Supervision Exercised

Collaborates with the Clinical Leader to provide input into the evaluation of the clinical practice of the staff.

Identifies and corrects factors contributing to problematic patient care.

Kathy A. Hausman
Department Level

[signature] MS RN CNAA.
Administrative Level

[signature]
Personnel

Rev. 11/17/93

FIGURE 1–1 *Continued*

Some medical record practitioners believe their coding and documentation expertise is valuable in maximizing reimbursement—one of the goals in a case management system. The issue of case management credentials depends on the case management model used. A clinically oriented model might require a nurse as a case manager, whereas a business-oriented model might benefit from a medical records or financial expert. In any case, the job description for the case manager should reflect the focus for the position (Fig. 1–1).

The third concern described in the literature about case management is how the manager is used. In some agencies every patient is assigned to a case manager who also provides total patient care. In other agencies the manager oversees care provided by other staff members for a group of patients. Another variation is the use of case managers as consultants when staff members have problems with patient care. These patients are often complex or outliers (not typical) within their diagnostic label.

Another dilemma associated with case management is how to develop and use clinical pathways. Clinical pathways guide care in a case management system. The focus of this book is on clinical pathways—their development, use, and evaluation.

CLINICAL PATHWAYS

A fairly recent term for case management—*outcomes management*—has been introduced to indicate the focus of health care on patient outcomes. Outcomes management also fits with the move in the United States for health care reform (St. Luke's Episcopal Hospital, 1994). The tools used by the health care team to identify patient outcomes are called *clinical pathways.*

Description of Clinical Pathways

Clinical pathways are also called *clinical paths, critical paths* or *pathways, care maps, collaborative plans of care, multidisciplinary action plans (MAPs), care paths,* and *anticipated recovery paths.* Some agencies have developed their own variation of the term, but the concept is essentially the same regardless of what term is used. This book uses the term *clinical pathways* to reflect their clinical nature and to avoid confusion for pathways used in the critical care setting.

Like the concept of case management, clinical pathways have been used in other fields for many years. The idea of standardizing care using patient protocols or routines was introduced into the health care literature more than 20 years ago. However, the environment was not receptive to the concept of clinical pathways until case management was introduced into the hospital setting.

Clinical pathways are interdisciplinary plans of care that outline the optimal sequencing and timing of interventions for patients with a particular diagnosis, procedure, or symptom. They are designed to minimize delays and use of resources while maximizing the quality of patient care. Thus clinical pathways are guidelines for care of patients who have a predictable course of illness, surgery, or event. They are typically developed for high-volume, high-cost, or high-risk diagnoses, procedures, or symptoms.

Features of Clinical Pathways

As is true with case management, everyone has his or her own idea about how to develop and use clinical pathways. Regardless of individual differences, pathways generally have four major features: patient outcomes, timeline, collaboration, and comprehensive aspects of care.

- *Patient outcomes.* Clinical pathways typically list expected patient outcomes by the time of discharge from the health care setting. For hospital use some pathways include both daily outcomes and discharge outcomes.
- *Timeline.* Clinical pathways usually contain specific timelines for sequencing interventions. In the hospital setting the typical time frame is day by day. However, for the emergency department and postanesthesia care unit the timeline may be hour by hour. In the rehabilitation or home setting the timeline may be week by week.
- *Collaboration.* Clinical pathways are jointly developed by multiple health care professionals, including the physician, and reflect interdisciplinary interventions.
- *Comprehensive aspects of care.* Clinical pathways track various aspects of care such as nutrition, diagnostic tests, treatments, medications, mobility and activity, patient teaching, and discharge planning. Many pathways begin with preadmission patient care, especially for elective procedures such as joint replacement or coronary artery bypass graft surgery.

Most experts in case management believe that not all patients are candidates for clinical pathways. The generic pathway is intended for the patient expected to progress along the timeline without experiencing complications. For more complex patients or those experiencing complications, use of clinical pathways may not be appropriate. However, some agencies have developed hybrid pathways for patients with these special needs.

Patients on clinical pathways typically have a case manager or case coordinator, who is usually a nurse. The case manager oversees and coordinates the patient's care and documents deviations from clinical pathways, called *variances.* Chapter 3 describes variance documentation and analysis in detail.

Benefits of Clinical Pathways

Clinical pathways can be very beneficial for the patient, physician and other health professionals, the health care agency, and third-party payors (Table 1–2).

TABLE 1–2 Benefits of Clinical Pathways

Patient	Health Team Members	Health Care Agency
Consumer involvement	Standardized, organized care	Supported by JCAHO
Patient education	Improved communication	Supported by third-party payors
Mutual goal setting	Reflection of current practice	Integration of quality improvement, utilization management, and risk management
Increased patient satisfaction	Increased staff satisfaction	Improved communication
	Educational tool for students and new graduates	Better competitive position
		Decreased length of stay
		Decreased costs
		Availability of data for evaluating care

Benefits for the Patient

As consumers of health care, patients should be involved in the care planning process. Until recently, most pathways were developed with very little input from patients. Often patients were not aware when they were on a pathway.

Some hospitals have recognized the value of patient involvement and have provided patients with a lay version of the pathway (see samples in Appendix A). By having lay pathways, patients know what care to expect and what the goals of care are. The pathway is also a teaching tool for the patient and family or significant others. Thus the primary benefits to the patient are improved customer satisfaction and mutual goal setting between the health care staff and the patient.

Benefits for Health Professionals

For physicians, clinical pathways provide a way to standardize and organize care for routine situations. Physicians within a group practice can use standard protocols to avoid confusion and inconsistencies in care. In addition, physicians can compare peer group practices with established guidelines.

For all health care professionals, care is coordinated and specified for improved communication among health team members. For example, a nurse caring for a postoperative total hip replacement patient can reinforce what the physical therapist has taught the patient about ambulation with a walker. Patient teaching can begin long before discharge so that the patient is prepared.

A written, interdisciplinary clinical pathway also helps to visualize current practice clearly; it indicates when either nothing is being done for the patient or too much is being done unnecessarily. Using pathways, nurses and other health professionals know what patient outcomes are expected in advance, thus improving collaboration and communication. Staff members who use clinical pathways as part of case management have reported increased job satisfaction, which decreases absenteeism and turnover (Cohen, 1991).

Students and new graduates in the health care professions can also benefit from clinical pathways. During their formal educational preparation, students are exposed to patients on an assigned day or for several days. They rarely follow a patient through the entire episode of illness or event. Clinical pathways teach students and new graduates how to carry out a comprehensive treatment plan in the most cost effective and timely manner; thus pathways can be teaching tools for both staff and patients by outlining the "big picture."

Benefits for the Health Care Agency

Clinical pathways have been used most often in hospitals. Their use in home care and other alternative health care settings has just begun. Clinical pathways can be very beneficial to a health care agency because of the following:

- The agency can demonstrate quality patient care to accrediting bodies (e.g., JCAHO) and licensing agencies.
- The agency is better able to negotiate contracts with managed care systems.
- The use of clinical pathways integrates quality improvement, utilization management, and risk management activities.
- Clinical pathways promote communication and delineate clearer expectations of care providers.
- The use of clinical pathways improves staff and patient satisfaction, thus improving the agency's competitive position.
- The use of clinical pathways decreases length of stay and thus saves money.

- Some third-party payors provide incentives or discounts to agencies that incorporate clinical pathways.
- Data are readily available for the evaluation of patient care by tracking variances and actual patient outcomes.

Benefits for Third-Party Payors

The primary benefit for third-party payors is that the insurers can establish standards to determine quality of care, outcomes, and reimbursement based on pathways. Health insurers clearly can determine what level of care is received for the reimbursement provided.

Potential Dilemmas Associated With Clinical Pathways

Although many hospitals and other health care agencies have or are developing clinical pathways, several areas of concern and controversy remain.

First, clinical pathways could be used as road maps for a plaintiff's attorney in medical malpractice claims, although they have not yet been tested (*Hospital Case Management,* February 1994). A pathway represents a standard to which the physician and other health care professionals are held accountable. Use of terms such as *variance,* a deviation from a pathway, suggests an error was made. An agency that uses pathways can minimize this liability by clarifying that the pathway is a *guideline* that must be flexible enough to individualize, depending on patient needs and responses. Agency policies and procedures should define what pathways are and when they should and should not be used.

Second, physicians may not actually use the pathways, even if they have input into their development. For example, after using pathways for 2 or 3 years, Alliant Health Systems' three hospitals in Louisville, Kentucky, found there was little physician use of the pathways (approximately 20% compliance) (*Hospital Case Management,* March 1993). Consequently, the hospital administration decided all clinical pathways must have intense physician involvement and there must be a system to measure pathway use and usefulness.

The new review process at Alliant resulted in ideal order sets, which included physician orders, nursing directives, and the basic elements of a treatment plan for a particular diagnosis. The physician must approve and activate the orders each day. This particular process is physician driven with some nurse involvement. Many agencies are opposed to physician-directed pathways because they are not collaborative in their development or use.

The third concern about clinical pathways as reported in the literature is the fear that there are inadequate data to demonstrate the value of pathways. Toronto Hospital in Canada found two factors affected the evaluation of pathways. First, there was no uniform, hospital-wide format for the various pathways, which made generating meaningful reports difficult. The second problem was the complex nature of variance analysis. Data were collected and tracked on 1200 patients using 300 clinical pathways. To help resolve this problem, the hospital began using an automated system to track data on its reformatted pathways (*Hospital Case Management,* March 1993).

Another dilemma is whether or not to place pathways on the medical record and, if so, where to place them. Most agencies include pathways as part of the permanent medical record. Some hospitals have put them within the physician's orders section, facilitating their use by physicians in planning care. Other agencies keep the pathways separate from the medical record and discard them after the patient is discharged.

If the pathway is additional paperwork that staff members are required to consult, a "throwaway" plan of care probably will not be used. The Kardex care plans of years past have shown that nurses and other health team members do not use this type of system.

Many experts believe that if the pathway is a part of the medical record, it should replace part of the existing documentation record. To accommodate this approach, some hospitals have combined patient care documentation with the pathway. In most cases only nurses document in this "charting-by-exception" method, although some agencies allow all disciplines to document on the pathways. Although it seems to avoid duplication, the charting-by-exception method as part of the pathway may not be accepted for fear of liability (*Critical Path Network,* May 1993; *Critical Path Network,* April 1994). However, the courts are beginning to recognize that the old adage, "If it wasn't documented, it wasn't done," is not always realistic.

The process of streamlining documentation yet documenting thoroughly is an unresolved dilemma. To address this concern, any agency that incorporates clinical pathways should include legal counsel on the pathway development team.

The Future of Clinical Pathways

In addition to addressing the dilemmas associated with clinical pathways, other questions must be answered. One of the most important issues is whether or not the pathway should cover the entire spectrum of care from preadmission through home care or other alternative care setting. A few hospitals have teamed with home care agencies to develop jointly comprehensive pathways. Some home health agencies are developing pathways independently. Examples are provided in Chapter 4.

Another issue is computerization of clinical pathways and variance analysis. Several software systems are currently available for tracking and coding data. For efficiency and accuracy, automation of clinical pathways is imperative. Chapter 3 discusses automation of variance analysis.

Data from case management and clinical pathways can also help to "cost out" specific health professional services such as nursing that have not traditionally been separate billable services. Comprising the largest department in a hospital setting, the costs and benefits associated with nursing services must be computed and analyzed. An automated system might track this information for the health care agency.

▼ CHAPTER HIGHLIGHTS ▼

- *Managed care* is generally an insurance-based term used to describe a system of health care delivery to control costs.
- Case management is a practice model that uses a systematic approach to identify high-cost patients and to manage patient care to ensure optimum outcomes.
- Case management is also called *care management, collaborative management, managed care, collaborative care,* or *outcomes management.*
- Some case management models are clinically oriented; some models are business oriented.
- Case managers are health care professionals, most often nurses, responsible for overseeing or providing the care for a group of patients.
- Case management saves money and improves the quality of patient care.

- Clinical pathways, also called *clinical paths, critical paths* or *pathways, care maps, collaborative plans of care, care paths,* and *anticipated recovery paths,* are interdisciplinary plans of care that outline the optimum sequencing and timing of interdisciplinary patient care for a particular diagnosis, procedure, or symptom.
- The four general features of clinical pathways are patient outcomes, a timeline, collaboration, and comprehensive aspects of care.
- Clinical pathways benefit the patient, the health care staff, the health care agency, and third-party payors.
- Deviations from clinical pathways are referred to as *variances,* which can be tracked by computer.

2

Development and Implementation of Clinical Pathways

As noted in Chapter 1, hospitals and other health care institutions are developing clinical pathways in response to healthcare reform issues at the state and federal level. Additionally, managed care companies and third-party payors are demanding documentation of a hospital's ability to provide quality care in a cost effective and efficient manner. Payors and other regulatory agencies are developing standards of care or practice guidelines with the expectation that physicians and hospitals will follow these standards for all aspects of patient care. However, pathways are never a substitute for clinical judgment and may be modified to meet the individual needs of the patient.

Clinical pathways, when developed through an interdisciplinary collaborative effort, provide clinicians with guidelines to coordinate, plan, implement, and monitor care to ensure that it is provided in a timely manner.

GETTING STARTED

Two key factors are necessary for the successful implementation of clinical pathways. First, the hospital's administrative team must support the concept of clinical pathways and provide the resources required to develop, implement, and evaluate the project (Wall and Proyect, 1994). Second, the project will advance more rapidly to completion if a person is appointed to champion the project through each stage of the developmental process. This person must have access to appropriate administrative authorities to guide the clinical pathway process.

Physician and staff "buy in" and input are vital to a successful project. Their cooperation will assist the hospital to meet its objectives and that of other agencies for resource utilization and achievement of an appropriate outcome for the patient's medical diagnosis and clinical condition. To obtain staff support for the project, the project should be announced to all staff. This can be accomplished through formal meetings, a notice on department bulletin boards, or the information (computer) system. A brief article should be placed in the hospital newsletter explaining the purpose, goals, and objectives of clinical pathways. Explain the benefits clinical pathways will bring to the patient, family, staff, and hospital. Be realistic about the problems and challenges that may be encountered.

TABLE 2–1   Clinical Pathway Education Guide

- Announcement of the project:
    - Definition and purpose of clinical pathway
    - Why the hospital will do it
    - Who the key players are
- Benefits and disadvantages of pathways for:
    - Patients
    - Families
    - Staff
    - Physicians
    - Hospital
    - Students

(NOTE: this information is often presented in an interview format.)

- General status update:
    - How staff can get involved
    - Roles and responsibilities of the staff
- Which pathway(s) were selected for initial implementation and where it will be piloted
- Format for pathway: call for staff input
- General review
- Implementation plan: schedule of in-services
- Evaluation of project
    - Variance analysis
    - Outcomes management

Set up a mechanism to inform all staff on a monthly basis about the status of the project. Explain how staff members can get involved and who they should contact for additional information about clinical pathways. Table 2–1 lists additional steps to take to educate the staff on clinical pathways.

Steering Committee

Once support is established for the development of clinical pathways, an interdisciplinary advisory team or steering committee is formed. Members are selected because of their interest, expertise, or leadership abilities. The steering committee leader must have the time and expertise to guide an interdisciplinary team and have a thorough understanding of the processes involved in project development and management. Communication and negotiation skills are essential as is the ability to move a project through an institution's approval mechanisms (Table 2–2).

Team members include physicians (attending and residents), nurses, and representatives from clinical departments (e.g., case management, dietary and food

TABLE 2–2   Qualities of Project Leader

Change agent

Creative

Excellent verbal and written communication skills

Experienced as a facilitator with demonstrated group processor skills

Negotiator

Team builder

Experience in program design and evaluation methodology
- Statistical analysis
- Data management

Well organized

TABLE 2–3   Project Team Member Areas

Admitting	Nursing
Case management	Pharmacy
Dietary and food services	Physician
Discharge planning	Quality improvement
Finance	Rehabilitation services
Information systems	Respiratory therapy
Laboratory	Social services
Materials management	Utilization review
Medical records	

This list is not all inclusive. Each institution should add additional staff according to its particular needs.

Some departments may be used to assist in the clinical pathway development on an "as needed" basis. The core group should consist of physicians, nurses, and personnel from other clinical departments applicable to the pathway under development.

services, respiratory therapy, rehabilitation services, social services, and utilization review). Representatives from materials management, laboratory, and pharmacy are equally important as part of the interdisciplinary team to determine alternative techniques that maintain patient care requirements for quality at a lesser cost. Other team members include someone from secretarial support, an information system specialist, and statistical support personnel. Staff input from medical records and finance areas is important to assist with data retrieval from the chart and other financial and utilization information (Table 2–3).

The quality improvement specialist's role is to provide the linkage of the quality improvement process with clinical management decision making. Through the use of objective data, the quality improvement specialist facilitates data analysis and decision making in the selection of which clinical pathway(s) to develop first.

Initial Steering Committee Meeting

The project leader calls the first meeting and sets a clear agenda. The meeting announcement includes a brief overview of the purpose, goals, and objectives of the project. A few articles or references about clinical pathways and examples from other hospitals provide each team member with an understanding of the nature and format of a pathway, thus minimizing the need to include an in-depth in-service presentation on clinical pathways at the first meeting. More detailed information about the application of clinical pathways for the particular setting can be presented at a later meeting.

The first meeting or two serve as orientation for the team members. The scope of the project, goals and objectives, and time table are reviewed, revised, and approved. The roles and responsibilities of the team members are discussed and agreed upon. The group may recommend the inclusion of additional team members, and some of the initial participants may elect to send a representative from their department who may have more expertise in the project or ability to meet the commitments of the project.

Steering Committee Responsibilities

General roles and responsibilities of the steering committee include the following:

- Establish format for meetings such as time, place, and need for agenda before meeting.

- Review roles of team members and identify a recorder (writes on board or flip chart), and secretary.
- Articulate purpose, goals, and objectives of the committee.
- Integrate continuous quality improvement or total quality management into pathway development.
- Obtain information needed to develop the pathway(s) (e.g., length of stay, cost, volume, problem prone or high-risk procedures).
- Recommend which pathways to develop first and prioritize the others.
- Develop guidelines for the format and use of the clinical pathway.
- Determine which departments need to participate or assist in pathway development.
- Advise hospital administration and other staff on project progress.
- Use practice pattern information, community standards, published guidelines, and comparisons to write pathway.
- Develop format to monitor variances
- Develop policies, procedures, and guidelines for use of clinical pathways.
- Develop an action plan to implement the clinical pathway(s).
- Evaluate the outcome of the project and make recommendations for the future.
- Assume accountability for the project.

Some hospitals have consulted with consumer and third-party payors to determine what they need and want from the care delivery system.

Pathway Team

In addition to the steering committee, many hospitals form subcommittees to develop the actual clinical pathway. The pathway teams develop the content of the clinical pathway. Group members include physicians, direct caregivers, staff members who are clinical experts in the diagnosis, and appropriate nonclinical staff (see Table 2–3). Throughout the process, the steering committee is available for administrative support and oversight for the project.

SELECTION OF THE CLINICAL PATHWAY

The clinical pathway selection process involves three steps: (1) selection of the target pathway; (2) establishment of the outcome(s) to achieve by using a clinical pathway for the target population; and (3) determination of the aspects of care to include in the pathway.

A number of factors influence which clinical pathways are developed initially (Wagie and Kraushar, 1994). The decision often is based on which diagnostic related group (DRG), international diagnostic code—9th edition (ICD-9 code), diagnostic test, or surgical procedure is high volume, high cost, high risk, or problem prone for the organization. This information may be obtained from a variety of sources. Financial reports provide information on the number of admissions according to DRG, average and targeted length of stay, and cost per admission. An additional source of information from the finance department is payment-denial letters from third-party payors such as Medicare or traditional insurance companies. Departmental and hospital-wide quality improvement activities may identify problem or high-risk diagnoses. DRGs that show high variability of practice patterns and difficulties with coordination of care may also be selected. Finally, many hospitals begin with those clinical pathways that have a high probability of successful implementation. Ultimately the goal is to select

TABLE 2–4 Decision Matrix

DRG	High Cost	High Volume	High Risk	Problem Prone	Changing Practice or Regulatory Guidelines
014	X	X	X	X	
209	X	X			X
121	X	X	X	X	X
198					X

DRGs that are high volume and create problems (however *problems* may be defined) for the hospital, particularly financial or length-of-stay issues.

The review of high-volume, high-cost, high-risk DRGs may show that there are many DRGs in these categories, and the team must select the most appropriate one to use for the clinical pathway (Table 2–4).

The methods and tools of continuous quality improvement can be applied to determine the most appropriate ones for the institution to use initially (Hofmann, 1993). A decision matrix can be made for each DRG regarding the number of admissions, length of stay, billable services, low reimbursement, and risk management cases (Table 2–5). Using the charts, the steering committee can compare each DRG by frequency, charge, and reimbursement. Another factor to consider is the level of interest expressed by the staff and physicians and the predictability of care requirements. If the staff members are interested in these pathways, they will be more willing to develop and use them.

Using the above information, the steering committee selects several diagnoses that appear problematic for the hospital. The use of force-field analysis may help the team members determine the priority for clinical pathway development (Table 2–6). Some hospitals choose to focus only on surgical case types, which are more likely to follow a standard clinical path. Unless a complication occurs, the patient's progress each day is predictable and easily monitored.

Developing a clinical pathway for a medical DRG is sometimes more difficult. In many cases the patient has other medical, psychosocial, or financial problems in addition to the primary diagnosis. Such a patient may exceed the recommended length of stay because of the impact of comorbidities. For example, a patient's primary diagnosis may be pneumonia, but he or she also is a diabetic in end-stage renal disease. Both the pneumonia and diabetic clinical pathways may be chosen,

TABLE 2–5 DRG Analysis Report

DRG	No. Cases	Average LOS	Targeted LOS	LOS Variance	Average Total Charge*	Average Payment*
143 (chest pain)	440	5.0	3.2	1.8	$3,600	$3,100
014 (CVA)	548	8.3	5.1	3.2	$6,058	$5,370
201 (total hip replacement)	411	6.5	5.2	1.3	$5,600	$3,430
296 (dehydration)	296	4.0	3.0	1.0	$1,200	$1,120
107 (CABG)	116	11.5	9.8	1.7	$12,000	$9,870
410 (chemotherapy	210	2.1	3.6	(.5)	$5,000	$4,700

LOS = length of stay; CVA = cerebrovascular accident; CABG = coronary artery bypass grafting.
*The dollar figures presented are for illustration purposes only.

TABLE 2–6   **Force-Field Analysis**

Driving Forces	Restraining Forces
Health care reform	Lack of information
Third-party payors	"Cookbook" medicine
Practice guidelines	Legal issues
Customer satisfaction	Risk management issues
Quality of care	Too much paperwork
	Lack of clinical information on usefulness

with careful attention given to avoiding duplication of diagnostic tests or procedures. Another option is to develop an uncomplicated and a complicated pathway for the same diagnosis. For example, this book contains clinical pathways for acute renal failure and renal failure with peritoneal dialysis. Clinical pathways for complicated and uncomplicated myocardial infarction are also included. Finally, based on clinical assessment, the physician may elect not to place the patient on any pathway.

Not all diagnoses that are problematic for the hospital should be resolved by developing a clinical pathway. Before making the final decision about which pathways to develop, the team should determine if the problem could be resolved using the methods and tools of quality improvement such as a flow chart or check sheet. Length of stay (LOS) may be longer than the norm because of type of patient seen in the hospital and the impact of socioeconomic factors on the patient and family. For example, some patients exceed LOS because a bed is not available in an extended care or rehabilitation facility. Others do not have the needed family support for earlier discharge. If this is the case, a clinical pathway will not resolve the issue and in fact may lead to an increased readmission rate. However, in some cases the use of a clinical pathway and variance reporting assists in identifying the root cause of the problem.

After the pathways to develop are selected, the steering committee identifies one or two broad goals to use to evaluate the usefulness of the clinical pathway. For example, the goal may be to reduce length of stay from 5 days to 3 days or to decrease cost by 5% without affecting quality of care.

DEVELOPING THE PATHWAY

The steering committee and pathway team meet to review sample pathways to determine the format to use to begin the actual writing of the clinical pathway for the hospital. A decision must be made whether the pathway is for inpatient use only or if it should cover the time before admission and after discharge. This decision will affect the categories selected for use on the pathway. The categories most often used are activity, consults, diagnostics, diet, discharge planning, laboratory tests, medications, teaching, and treatments. Expected outcomes may be included as an aspect of care each day or may be listed as overall outcomes for the particular diagnosis. (See Chapter 5 for the format used in this book.)

Next the members of the pathway teams review medical records specific for the selected DRG or ICD-9 code to analyze practice patterns and to determine how many procedures and laboratory tests are done for each designated diagnosis. Information about the number of admissions, length of stay, and cost by case is obtained from the finance department in collaboration with the information services staff. Data are collected to identify common orders, timing of interventions, nursing care, and other necessary information such as use of diagnostic and laboratory tests and supplies. All this information is reviewed to determine if it is necessary and if there is a more effective way to achieve the same results. For example, laboratory and diagnostic turn-around times and medication delivery time are reviewed to see if they can be reduced or if there are barriers to more timely delivery of care. When feasible, the team should compare physicians within the hospital, looking for those with the best demonstrated clinical outcomes to use in developing the medical components of the pathway.

Clinical pathways are based on sound clinical research, published guidelines, and a review of the literature. The clinical indicators in JCAHO's IMSystem is an additional source of information. Beginning in 1995, participating hospitals will receive comparative information concerning specific quality indicators or important aspects of obstetric, perioperative, cardiovascular, oncology, and trauma care. The hospitals will be able to compare their performance to that of all other participants, knowing that all participants are collecting the same data and have indicator rates calculated the same way. Although participation in this program is voluntary at this time, it will be required in the future after beta testing is completed and appropriate revisions have been made to the system. Because the IMSystem is in the testing stage, most experts agree that at this time the indicators should be used only if they fit with the hospital's priorities (*Hospital Case Management,* June 1994).

The team meets to discuss best practices and to refer to information from other health care facilities that have used pathways. The data are compared to national and state norms to identify those that typically exceed the norm. The team may suggest modifications or changes in current practice patterns based on a detailed analysis of the information collected.

The initial goal is to develop the ideal clinical pathway that will address the needs of the majority of the patients who will be followed on the pathway. Using brainstorming techniques and incorporating the information obtained as described earlier, the draft pathway is reviewed for improvement opportunities. Subgroups may be needed to work on identified issues or opportunities. Revisions to the pathway may be recommended by the team after they have had experience placing information into the categories selected. As noted previously, interdisciplinary involvement is critical to the successful implementation of a clinical pathway.

Terminology used on the path must be easily understood by the interdisciplinary team that will care for the patient. Only hospital-approved abbreviations should be used, and the use of jargon should be eliminated.

At times clinical pathways fail because of lack of physician involvement. As with other staff members, physicians must be involved in the process from the beginning. They should be provided with information about the benefits they and their patients will receive (Merry, 1994). Physicians may be reluctant to use clinical pathways because of fears that hospitals and insurance companies will dictate how they are to practice medicine.

Providing physicians with information about their own specific practice pattern may help gather their support. First, working with several physicians, the ideal practice pattern is developed (*Hospital Case Management,* July 1994). These practice guidelines may be based on the guidelines developed by professional societies, regulatory agencies, or published guidelines such as those written by the Agency for Healthcare Policy and Research. Next, each physician's own practice pattern for the particular diagnosis is measured against the ideal standard and for direct costs and length of stay. Costs are reviewed in more detail, particularly

TABLE 2-7 Guidelines to Obtain Physician Support

1. Involve the physician in the process from the beginning:
   a. Clinical pathway to pilot
   b. Format to use
   c. Material to include on pathway
2. Show benefits to patient and family.
3. Demonstrate benefits to the physician's personal practice.
4. Use objective data to provide the physician with his or her practice pattern information and how it compares to that of other physicians in the hospital and community.
5. As needed, assist the physician to change or modify practice pattern based on community standards, guidelines, etc.
6. Share variance analysis data.
7. Elicit the physician's involvement and support to review and revise the pathway based on variance data and changes in practice guidelines or technology.
8. Follow-up on agreed action plan or strategies for doing things better.
9. KEEP THE LINES OF COMMUNICATION OPEN.

for tests and procedures if there is high variability. Another opportunity to increase physician involvement is to track adherence to the clinical pathway and report variance directly to the involved physician. Physicians are accustomed to making decisions based on scientific evidence and objective data. By showing them in a concise and timely manner how variations in their practice pattern are unnecessarily costly and that reducing variation in practice will not compromise patient care, they should respond in a positive manner. Table 2–7 provides additional information on strategies to use to obtain physician support for clinical pathway projects (*Hospital Case Management*, November 1994).

Final Path Check

Before its submission for the hospital approval process, the pathway should be reviewed to determine if everything is there that should be and if anything can be eliminated to save cost and decrease length of stay without compromising quality of care. The pathway is reviewed for appropriateness by all involved disciplines and should not be only a physician and nursing document. Clinical expert review of the pathway for compliance with or exceeding the standards of care for community and other regulatory agencies is a necessary final step.

At this time consideration is given to what and how variances will be monitored and outcomes evaluated. An outcome describes the end result of patient care, an improvement in the patient's condition, or a complete resolution of the patient's medical problem (e.g., the patient is expected to demonstrate the correct usage of the metered dose inhaler).

The pathway-specific team writes the clinical pathway and includes the outcome statement(s). The team selects those aspects of care that, if not followed, will lead to the patient's not achieving the expected outcome.

Guidelines, policies, or procedures for the use of the pathway within the hospital are reviewed for clarity of content and consistency. Policies are written about how the pathway should be followed and how variances are monitored and documented. An implementation and evaluation action plan is prepared.

Finally, the clinical pathway should be reviewed for legal and risk management purposes. The pathway must be consistent with the rules and regulation of local, state, and federal regulatory agencies and accreditation bodies. Documentation is maintained about which attending and consulting physicians gave their approval for the use of a particular clinical pathway.

IMPLEMENTATION

The introduction of clinical pathways is not easy. Changing practice patterns require people to change the way they have been caring for their patients. It is important to be sensitive to the problems that the staff may have with the change (Lucas, 1994). Help them understand the need for the change. Listen to their concerns and involve them every step of the way. Whenever someone expresses enthusiasm for the project, get him or her involved in literature review, chart review, developing or reviewing a clinical pathway, and implementing the pathway. Ask for his or her opinion, and find out what he or she fears most about clinical pathway implementation. Recognize that the staff members may be concerned that they do not have the knowledge base, skills, or information on how to follow and use the clinical pathway. Provide reassurance that the required in-service education will be done to enable their success. Include information on change management, teams and team work, interprofessional relationships, accountability, and professional practice.

Departments directly affected by the pathway need more information than those with limited interaction. Regardless of the level of use of the pathway, all staff must be aware of the purpose and correct use of the clinical pathway and how it improves the clinical care of the patient and family. Staff must be aware that the pathways are not standing orders unless specified by hospital policy. The physician may elect to use or modify a clinical pathway based on the patient's clinical condition.

Resource staff must be available on all shifts for the first few weeks of implementation. During the first 3 or 4 days, staff members who have the educational background to answer questions that arise as implementation of the pathways begins should be physically present in the hospital. After this time, availability by beeper is generally sufficient.

It is best to start with only one or two pathways, which then are used on a pilot basis on the appropriate patient care area. Until the clinical pathway has actually been followed on several patients, it is not known how well it will meet patient outcomes and the objectives of the staff and hospital. Time is needed to evaluate the pathway's effectiveness and to obtain input from the staff on how it could be done better. Within 3 to 6 months, sufficient numbers of patients should have been followed using the pathway, and changes to it can be made based on the objective data collected.

HOW TO USE PATHWAYS

The clinical pathway is most often placed in the physician order's section of the patient's medical record, the nursing or medication Kardex, or at the patient's bedside. The clinical pathway may also be placed in a separate binder used by the case manager or primary nurse and other members of the interdisciplinary team. Depending on hospital policy or guidelines, the physician may order that the pathway is followed as written, modified, or not followed at all.

The clinical pathway is reviewed by the caregivers or case manager or both at the start of each shift and throughout the day to evaluate the patient's progress toward the day's expected outcomes. Deviation or variance from the listed patient care activity is documented and an action plan developed by the interdisciplinary team to resolve the problem. More information on variance analysis and evaluation is presented in Chapter 3.

Each hospital must define for itself the best way to document the patient's progress in meeting the outcomes for clinical pathway protocols. This may be done

TABLE 2–8 Clinical Pathway Program

1. Educate and obtain support from staff and physicians.
2. Form the interdisciplinary teams:
    a. Steering committee and pathway-specific group
    b. Group to identify potential obstacles to implementation
3. Data collection: determine patient population, DRG, ICD-9 code to focus on those who are:
    a. High volume
    b. High cost
    c. High risk
    d. Difficult to manage
4. Use continuous quality improvement methods and tools to select:
    a. Pareto charts
    b. Statistical process control chart
5. Determine which ICD-9 code is most predictable.
6. Determine staff interest.
7. Select pathways to develop.
8. Develop format for pathway.
9. Select interdisciplinary clinical experts for pathway team.
10. Collect clinical pathway data:
    a. Medical record review for practice patterns
    b. Literature review
    c. Comparison with other institutions
    d. Practice guidelines
11. Write the pathway:
    a. Review by staff
    b. Review as necessary
12. Develop variance analysis system:
    a. Information needed to measure compliance with the pathway
    b. Outcomes measurement
    c. Clinical and financial measurements
13. Present pathway to hospital committees for approval: incorporate revision.
14. Develop implementation plan.
15. Provide in-service staff.
16. Use pilot pathway for 3 to 6 months; revise as needed.
17. Monitor variances:
    a. Develop automated data collection if possible
    b. Present variance data to staff and physicians

directly on the pathway, on the back of the pathway, or in the progress notes. The important point is that the clinical pathway becomes part of the patient's permanent medical record and that the patient's progress is consistently documented on the chart.

Using the clinical pathway as a documentation tool is not without risk. As with any charting system, the old adage "if it's not documented, it's not done" may apply (*Hospital Case Management,* February 1994). If documentation is done directly on the pathway, enough space for the signature of the person accountable for following the pathway and one for the nurse providing patient care should be available. Written policies and procedures or guidelines indicating how and when the pathway should and should not be used must be in place. The policy should include direction for how and where to document deviation from the clinical pathway. Additionally, a record should be kept of who developed the pathway and who approved its use.

This chapter has provided a brief overview of the steps needed to develop and implement clinical pathways (Table 2–8). Refer to the reference list for more detailed information on clinical pathway development.

▼ **CHAPTER HIGHLIGHTS** ▼

- Two key factors are necessary for the successful implementation of clinical pathways:
    Administrative support
    Staff member who will champion the project through each stage of the process
- The principles of the change theory are used to assist the staff to change their practice patterns.
- In-service education begins early in the planning stages of clinical pathways.
- An interdisciplinary team implements the project.
- Steps to implement clinical pathways are outlined on Table 2–8.
- Obtaining physician support is important early in the development of pathways.
- A steering committee provides administrative oversight, selects the pathways to implement, and devises the evaluation system.
- Clinical pathways are usually selected based on the following criteria:
    High-volume, high-cost, high-risk procedures
    Problem-prone procedures
    Insurance denials
    Quality improvement initiatives
- The methods and tools of continuous quality improvement are used to determine the most appropriate pathways to develop.
- The pathway-specific team develops the content of the clinical pathway.
- Variance analysis data are collected, analyzed, and reviewed for needed action.

3

Variance Analysis and Evaluation

An important component of the clinical pathway process is outcome evaluation. Although the format for writing expected outcomes varies, it is defined or described as the end result of care or the outcome the patient should demonstrate by discharge. Some institutions include a daily outcome statement as part of the category or aspect of care column on the clinical pathway. Other institutions list two or three overall expected patient outcomes based on the medical diagnosis. Each day or at discharge, the case manager reviews the clinical pathway or medical record or both. Information is obtained to determine whether or not the patient has met the defined outcome. If a variance has occurred, it is documented in the required format.

VARIANCE

If the expected outcome has not been met, variance data are reviewed. A variance is the difference between what is expected and what actually happened or occurred. It is a deviation from an activity in any of the categories or key aspects of care listed on the clinical pathway that potentially affects the expected outcome for the patient. As stated in Chapter 2, variance monitoring is performed to determine if patient outcomes or planned results occur on a consistent basis. Variance analysis consists of carefully reviewing the data for trends and developing and implementing an action plan to respond to identified problems.

Variances may be positive or negative, depending on the clinical situation (Acord-Szczesny, 1994). For example, a positive variance occurs when a patient progresses more rapidly toward the expected outcome and is discharged earlier than expected. A negative variance occurs when the activities on the clinical pathway are not completed within the designated time frame and length of stay is prolonged, costs are higher than expected, or the patient does not meet the expected outcome, regardless of the reason. Trends in both positive and negative variances should be reviewed and acted upon.

Causes of Variance

Many hospitals identify the cause of variances as (1) hospital or system; (2) clinician or caregiver; (3) patient or family; or (4) community related (Table 3–1). Under each of these headings is a list of why the problem may have occurred. For coding purposes, a code number or short abbreviation is assigned to each cause. A

TABLE 3–1 Variance Documentation

DRG No. _____ Length of Stay _____

Medical Record No.	Actual LOS	Patient/Family Related	System Related	Caregiver Related	Community Related	Comments

HOSPITAL/SYSTEM RELATED
01 Department (specify)
  a. Delay, prolonged wait
  b. Omission
  c. Incorrect
  d. Results not in
  e. Not completed
02 Bed not available
03 Bed not clean
04 OR change
05 Department not open on weekends
06 Equipment missing/not available
07 Records not available for discharge or transfer
08 Insurance-related problem
09 Other

CAREGIVER RELATED
01 History and physical
02 Assessment
03 Orders
04 Consent
05 Medication
06 Education
07 Procedure, interventions
08 IV lines
09 Consult
  a. Delay notifying
  b. Delay seeing
10 MD
  a. Delay notifying
  b. Delay seeing
  c. Delay orders
  d. Delay procedures
11 Anesthesiology delay
12 RN delay
13 Incomplete documentation (Admission assessment, data base, flow sheet, discharge plan)
14 Deviation from pathway not addressed within appropriate time frame
15 Transcription error
16 Incomplete records
17 Other

PATIENT/FAMILY RELATED
01 NPO
02 Allergies
03 Patient complications: Specify _____
04 Patient complications: Infection _____
05 Readmission within 30 days
06 Refused procedure
07 Suspected/confirmed infection
08 Pain
09 Mobility limitations
10 GI (e.g., nausea, vomiting)
11 Delay in decision making by patient/family
12 Lack of family support
13 Financial issues
14 Insurance issues
15 Other

COMMUNITY RELATED
01 Delay transfer
02 Bed not available
  a. Extended care
  b. Rehabilitation
  c. Long-term care
03 Ambulance
04 Home health/VNA
05 Home modification
06 Equipment
  a. Medical (ventilator)
  b. Adaptive/assistive

heading for "special causes" or one-time events may also be included. A limitation of this system is that it shows what happened but not why the variance occurred.

Hospital or system failures occur because of inefficient hospital operations and often require administrative action to resolve. Examples of this type of failure include a test or procedure not performed on the specified day, a prolonged wait for service, or a bed not being available.

Caregiver variances are due to staff-related issues, including treatments not completed, patient education not done, or incomplete documentation.

At times variances occur because of patient- or family-related issues such as complications of hospitalization or because the patient refuses a particular procedure or test.

Community variances are also referred to as external hospital-related variances. External system failures may be due to lack of bed availability in an extended care or rehabilitation facility or lack of availability of home care.

TABLE 3–2   **Variance Documentation: Free Text**

Patient: _____

Date of admission: _____

Diagnosis: _____

Date	Variance	Reason	Comments/ Action Plan	Signature

Additionally, variances may occur as a one-time incident or a special cause (*Hospital Case Management,* August 1993). For example, x-ray procedures may be delayed or canceled one day because of a large number of patients in the emergency department secondary to a bus or train crash. Finally, a variance may occur secondary to changes in the patient's health status or because of a complication of chronic medical conditions not associated with the reason for the current admission.

To address a limitation of the previously discussed coding system of variance monitoring, some hospitals use an open or free text tool (Table 3–2). With this system, the type of variance and the reason for its occurrence are written in the assigned columns. A comment section or section for an action plan is also included.

DATA COLLECTION

Care must be taken to collect only data that reflect the key aspects of the treatment process. Questions the team may want to consider when determining the data elements to monitor are given in Table 3–3. Key aspects of care are those critical to the patient's outcome. They include diagnostic procedures, laboratory tests, nursing interventions, and other monitoring activities. One way to determine if the element is a key aspect is to ask, "What would happen or what would the effect be on outcome (including quality of care and life and financial outcome) if this element were omitted or delayed?" (Miller, 1994). Be sure to obtain agreement from the clinical staff on what the key aspects of care are. Typical collected data include outcome information, cost and financial data, and descriptive data such as length of stay (Table 3–4).

Variance monitoring can be labor intensive. Too often a hospital attempts to monitor so many aspects of care that it leads to analysis paralysis. In other words, so much data are collected that sophisticated analysis techniques are required to make any sense of them. Too much data can lead to significant variances being

TABLE 3–3   Variance Monitoring: Questions to Ask

1. What data elements should be monitored
   Key aspects of care
   Critical incidents
2. What is the impact on outcome or quality of care if the data element is omitted?
3. Can the data be collected?
   How easily?
   Where are data located?
4. What format will be used to collect the data?
   Manual: who develops and prints the forms?
   Automated:
     Hardware requirements
     Software availability
     Cost
5. Who will collect the data? What training is required?
6. How and who will perform the data analysis?
   Quality Improvement Council
   Case managers
   Steering committee
   Pathway team
7. What will be done with the information?
   Action plan
   Additional education
   Review or revise clinical pathway
   Change in practice pattern
8. Who is responsible for seeing that follow-up activities are completed?
9. What will be done if the agreed-on action plan is not followed?

missed because the information is buried under the avalanche of minutia. Monitoring variance data that are difficult to collect or that require the use of extensive resources such as computer software programs is another problem that may be encountered.

Chart Review

The patient's chart is reviewed to determine if and why a variance occurred. Variance analysis may be done concurrently or retrospectively. Concurrent data or daily collection of variance information is performed when the clinical pathway is used to direct the day-to-day clinical care of the patient and is considered a permanent part of the medical record. Continuous review of the clinical pathway may also be done to meet payor requirements, to ensure that a pathway is being followed, and to ensure documentation occurs according to hospital policy or guidelines.

TABLE 3–4   Key Aspects of Care: DRG or ICD-9 Code

1. Outcome information
   Discharge disposition (home, extended care facility)
   Status at discharge
2. Financial data
   Average total charges
   Average cost per day
   Variable cost per day
3. Descriptive data
   Average length of stay (ALOS)
   Targeted length of stay (TLOS)
   Number of patients in each pathway

Retrospective analysis is generally done to compare outcomes of different patients followed on the same clinical pathway. This information is used to determine whether or not the pathway should be reviewed, revised, and updated. It may also show that the staff members need additional help to comply with hospital policy.

Data may be collected and analyzed by the case manager or any other staff member with the needed skills. After the data have been statistically analyzed, the information is organized in a readable format and presented to the medical staff, members of the pathway specific team, quality improvement council, case managers, and others as determined by hospital guidelines.

Automated Systems

A small number of hospitals have purchased or developed software packages to automate clinical pathways and data management. Before any hospital or other health care agency makes this high-cost investment, several elements of the case management and clinical pathway system need to be in place. First, the agency must have a well-defined clinical pathway process that has been tested and successfully used for a period of time. Second, adequate personnel and other resources need to be available for learning and using the automated system. Finally, the agency needs to demonstrate that what it is doing with clinical pathways has improved the quality of patient care.

Once the decision to automate has been made, the agency needs to examine whether the new software can interface with the current hospital information system. A number of large information system vendors have developed or are developing software packages that link with their current systems. Some systems are still in the beta testing phase of development.

Other vendors are developing software that can be integrated into electronic patient records. CareMinder, from TDS Healthcare Systems Corporation, has a full spectrum of use for case managers, including clinical pathways and flow sheets for documentation. This system requires bedside terminals. PACE (Patient Care Expert System) provides a computer-based patient record without the high cost of bedside terminals. Table 3–5 lists some of the automated systems available for clinical pathways and data management. Any system that the agency purchases should do more than merely print clinical pathways.

Staff members generally find that their work is more efficient when data are managed through an automated or computerized system. A major advantage of automation, then, is the ability to analyze large amounts of data statistically in a short period of time. It also provides consistency in the data collection format, analysis of data input, and final report printout.

TABLE 3–5 **Examples of Automated Data Bases for Clinical Pathways and Case Management**

Software Package	Vendor
Case Trakker	IMA Technologies
Outcome	Evaluation Systems International
CareMinder	TDS Healthcare Systems Corporation
PACE	Health Care Expert Systems, Inc.
ACT/PC	ACT/PC

Currently, the greatest disadvantages of most automated systems are the cost of hardware and software and the amount of staff time needed to learn how to use the system. Some systems may require more time to capture the data and input it into the system than if it were done manually.

DATA ANALYSIS

Variances that consistently occur on a clinical pathway that has been followed on a variety of patients are thoroughly analyzed. The interdisciplinary team uses the methods and tools (e.g., flow charts, brainstorming) of quality improvement to identify the root cause(s) of the variance. Considered information includes the cost, average length of stay, readmission rates, and other key indicators (e.g., laboratory and diagnostic tests) associated with the pathway. The team makes a recommendation to change the process or timing of activities within the pathway. The team may find that the pathway must be totally rewritten after additional information is obtained through a review of the literature, comparison with other hospitals, and identification of changes in practice patterns, technology, or research.

Other information to evaluate includes the staff's and physicians' response to the clinical pathway. Do they understand how to use the pathway? Are they aware of the benefits for the patient, their families, the hospital, and themselves? The team seeks staff input into changes or revisions of policies or guidelines to make it easier to use the clinical pathway appropriately. For example, is the pathway easily accessible for the staff to use; is the information easy to read; is it relevant to their practice? Another reason the pathway may not be followed is that the particular patient population for the pathway has significant comorbidities such as diabetes and chronic airflow limitation.

ACTION PLAN

The final step of variance monitoring and variance analysis is to develop an action plan to correct the identified problems. The plan of action is documented and includes the name(s) of the person responsible for ensuring the action is taken and the date the changes should be complete. This information is referred to the quality improvement staff who monitor's the plan and ensures that the required improvements are made.

This chapter has provided a brief overview of the various components of variance monitoring and evaluation. Refer to the reference list for more information on variance analysis.

▼ CHAPTER HIGHLIGHTS ▼

- A variance is the difference between what is expected and what actually occurs.
- Variance analysis consists of reviewing the data for trends and developing and implementing an action plan to respond to identified problems.
- Variances may be positive or negative.
- Causes of variances are hospital or system, clinician or caregiver, patient or family, and community related.
- Data collected for variance monitoring reflect key aspects of care such as medication administration, laboratory findings, and length of stay.
- Concurrent variance monitoring is done when the clinical pathway is used to direct the daily care of the patient.

- Retrospective variance monitoring is done to compare outcomes of treatment of different patients followed on the same clinical pathway.
- As a result of variance analysis, the clinical pathway may be modified or completely changed, or the staff may be given additional education.

4

Use of Clinical Pathways in a Variety of Health Care Settings

The generic clinical pathways in this book focus on adult medical-surgical and critical care health problems seen in the acute care setting. However, in some hospitals pathways have become so useful that they are being developed for specialty units such as psychiatry, labor and delivery, and pediatrics. Additionally, pathways using varying timelines are being implemented in settings other than hospitals. This chapter describes some of the creative ways that clinical pathways are used throughout the United States to provide quality care while maintaining cost control.

USE OF CLINICAL PATHWAYS IN HOSPITAL SPECIALTY UNITS

Most clinical pathways published to date are designed for adult medical-surgical diagnoses, although some hospitals have developed pathways to meet the special needs for other areas of medicine. For example, several West Coast hospitals have been using psychiatric diagnoses on pathways in their acute psychiatric units for several years. At St. Joseph's Hospital and Health Care Center in Tacoma, Washington, overall length of stay (LOS) dropped from $8\frac{1}{2}$ days before using psychiatric pathways to $4\frac{1}{2}$ days after beginning to use pathways (*Hospital Case Management,* October 1993). Examples of diagnoses for which clinical pathways have been developed at St. Joseph's institution include major depression, dementia, substance abuse and chemical dependency, and personality disorder.

At Hemet Valley Medical Center in Southern California, Multidisciplinary Action Plans (MAPs) have been developed for depression, organic brain syndrome, schizophrenia, schizo-affective disorder, and bipolar affective disorder—high-volume psychiatric diagnoses. Each pathway is divided into aspects of care such as nutrition, medication, diagnostic studies, patient education, and discharge planning.

Clinical pathways are also being used in perioperative areas. The perioperative staff may participate on interdisciplinary committees to develop pathways for surgical DRGs or to design pathways for ambulatory surgery. Some operating room (OR) managers are also using pathways to reduce and standardize supplies, especially for high-volume, predictable surgeries such as total hip replacement. Supply vendors are working with OR management on this type of inventory system (Patterson, 1994).

Covenant Medical Center

Waterloo, IA

ASU Critical Pathway

Eye Procedures

Exp. Time: 60 minutes

	Initial	15 Minutes	30 Minutes	60 Minutes	120 Minutes	180 Minutes
Discharge Planning	Let patient and family know the approximate length of stay is 1 hour.	Go over Dr. _____ discharge instructions before Dr. _____ comes to see the patient.	Give discharge instructions to patient and family. Be sure to send home ID card, tape, prescriptions, sunglasses, eye shield and medications.			
Key Nursing Activities/ Teaching	1. Temperature, pulse, respirations and blood pressure as routine. 2. Assess drainage from eye. 3. Assess pain and offer medication if needed. 4. Observe for nausea and vomiting. 5. Offer liquid as tolerated. 6. Elevate head of bed 60 degrees if local, 45 degrees if general. 7. Be sure order is to pharmacy to get medication labeled. 8. Assess IV site and rate.	Continue to assess #1–#5, #8. Discontinue IV if tolerating liquids by mouth. Elevate head of bed 60 to 90 degrees.	Continue to assess #1–#5, #8. Assist with getting dressed, if needed. Assess pain relief if medication given. Up in chair.	Continue to asseses #1–#5, #8 Discharge.		
Key Patient Activities/ Outcome	Patient will tolerate head of bed elevated 40 to 60 degrees. Patient will take liquids without nausea.	Patient will tolerate head of bed elevated 90 degrees. Patient will tolerate liquids.	Patient will be dressed for discharge.	Patient or family will verbalize understanding of discharge instructions. Will tolerate sitting up in chair. Will have taken 1 glass of liquid. Will not have severe eye pain.		

FIGURE 4–1 Example of a clinical pathway used in ambulatory surgery. Developed by the Ambulatory Surgery Staff, Covenant Medical Center, Waterloo IA 50702. Adapted from CareMap® System, The Center for Case Management.)

At Baptist Memorial Hospital and Baptist Memorial Hospital–East in Memphis, Tennessee, perioperative case managers work to prevent delays or cancellations in surgical procedures. Their clinical pathways for 1-day (same day) surgery use "phases" as the timeline, including the preoperative phase, intraoperative phase, postanesthetic care unit (PACU) phase, and postoperative follow-up.

USE OF DIFFERENT TIMELINES FOR CLINICAL PATHWAYS

As mentioned previously, the usual daily timelines on most pathways are not appropriate for all settings. For example, same-day surgical settings often map their pathways by minutes or hours. Figure 4–1 illustrates a pathway for eye procedures developed by the ambulatory surgery staff at the Covenant Medical Center in Waterloo, Iowa. This pathway follows the care of the patient during the 60 minutes through the procedure and follow-up. Patient outcomes are listed for each time interval. A major benefit of ambulatory pathways is that they can be used both as part of nursing orientation and for direction for patient care.

Another setting within the hospital in which minutes, hours, or intervals may be used as the timeline is the emergency department (ED). At Mercy Hospital in Toledo, Ohio, diabetic patients were the first group targeted for clinical pathways. The diabetic patient experiencing ketoacidosis (DKA) is typically admitted through the ED and transferred to a general unit or critical care between hours 2 and 3. This pathway for the patient with DKA is referred to as a *clinical progression* because it tracks the patient from one part of the hospital to another (*Hospital Case Management*, February 1993).

USE OF PATHWAYS THAT TRACK THE CONTINUUM OF CARE

JCAHO's 1995 standards stress requirements for multidisciplinary collaboration and the continuum of care. Highlights of the chapter, "Continuum of Care," of the JCAHO accreditation manual are found in Table 4–1. The use of clinical pathways can help hospitals meet these standards.

One approach to mapping patient care across the entire continuum of care is shown in Figure 4–2 for patients receiving chemotherapy. At the University of California at Davis Medical Center, ovarian cancer patients (stages III and IV) receive complex dose-intensive chemotherapy regimens that require careful coor-

TABLE 4–1 Highlights of JCAHO Continuum of Care Requirements for 1995

- Have a process to facilitate patients' access to the appropriate clinical service and caregiver(s), based on assessed need.
- Perform an assessment before accepting patients into a given service or setting.
- Ensure as part of the admissions process that patients and families are appropriately informed about the care that will be provided.
- Assure continuity of care—a logical progression of service from assessment and diagnosis through planning and treatment.
- Assure that all care is coordinated by the health professionals in the various settings.
- Refer, transfer, or discharge the patient to the appropriate provider if assessment data indicate that a patient needs another level of care.
- Consider all the patient's care needs in the discharge plan to assure continuity of care.
- Make sure there is an exchange of appropriate patient and clinical information when patients are admitted, referred, transferred, or discharged.
- Assure that decisions to provide or deny care or service are based on the needs of the patient.

Collaborative Path Ovarian Cancer

Date/Cycle	Day 1/Cycle 1	Day 8/Cycle 1	Week Three/Cycle 1	Week Four/Cycle 1
Setting	Cancer Center Clinic/IV infusion center	Inpatient Unit	Home	Home
Key Nursing Activities	Begin new patient teaching: Routine and Schedule of tx Protocol. Teach chemotherapy toxicity's per chemotherapy teaching protocol, self-care and G-CSF if started cycle 1. Evaluate need for Venous Access Device (VAD). Tour IV infusion. Initiate discharge plan for home care if pt. starts G-CSF or has new VAD.	Review chemotherapy toxicity's, self-care, blood counts, and G-CSF teaching. Reinforce how to access system for side effects and teach role of hospital team. Initiate discharge plan for home care. Teach home antiemetic administration. Evaluate need for VAD and teach care of line if needed. **Note: If no home health referral made, pt. must be able to do all activities week 3 and 4 as self-care.**	Assess to S/SX of chemotherapy toxicity; specifically pancytopenia, nausea and vomiting, dehydration and electrolyte imbalance. Draw lab work. Monitor and teach G-CSF injection. Evaluate need for VAD and teach care of line if needed. Frequency BIW X 2 then weekly X 2. If on G-CSF or new central line, daily until competent then as above.	Same as week 3
Treatment plan coordination	Set up IV infusion appointments. Submit HAR for hospital admission. Orders written for Day 1 and 8 and sent to IV infusion. Arrange for shadow file transfer to inpt.	Hospital admission for Cis-Platinum. Arrange for shadow file and discharge instruction sheet transfer back to clinic. Initiate home care plan if not started in clinic.	Review calendar with pt. and primary nurse.	Same as week 4. Arrange to have preadmission lab work ready prior to clinic visit.
Labs/tests	CBC, CA 125, Chem 20 CBC BIW if on GCSF	Day 7 CBC, Chem 7, Mg+	CBC BIW if on GCSF if not CBC weekly, Mg+, Chem 7 Day 21	CBC same as week 3
Chemotherapy	Carboplatin Cytoxan	CisPlatin		
G-CSF	Day 2–7 if started first cycle. Note: may be started after neutropenia develops.	Day 10–15	Day 15–17 eval counts for need to continue.	
Self-care	G-CSF (if nec.), VAD (if nec.) management of N/V, prevention of dehydration.	Same as week 1	Same as week 1, prevention of infection and bleeding.	Same as week 3
Consults	MSW outpt CNS if high risk Discharge planner	MSW inpt CNS if high risk Discharge planner		

FIGURE 4–2 Example of a clinical pathway reflecting the continuum of care. (Courtesy of Patti Palmer, RN, MS, OCN, and Oncology Nursing Leadership Group: University of California, Davis Medical Center and University of California, Davis Cancer

dination between the inpatient and ambulatory care settings. The pathway takes the patient from the Cancer Center–IV Infusion Center to the hospital, then to the home setting, for care over a period of many weeks.

Many hospital-based and freestanding rehabilitation programs are also using clinical pathways that "move" the patient from the hospital to rehabilitation to ambulatory or home-based care. At the Legacy Rehabilitation Services and Extended Care Facilities in Portland, Oregon, clinical pathways reduce LOS while providing coordinated patient services. Charting by exception has been incorporated into the pathways to save staff time as well (*Hospital Case Management,* January 1994).

Emory University Hospital in Atlanta has developed pathways for head-injury patients from admission through rehabilitation that can be used as a general guideline for care and individualized as needed. Some complex trauma patients admitted for rehabilitation must be on two or more pathways concurrently (*Hospital Case Management,* January 1994).

USE OF PATHWAYS IN ALTERNATE CARE SETTINGS

Most clinical pathways are designed for use in the hospital or from hospital admission through home care. Both home health and long-term care settings are beginning to develop their own pathways. Clinical pathways are often more difficult to design for these settings because care is not as predictable as in the hospital. In addition, many of the patients in home health and long-term care have multiple diagnoses; many of these diagnoses are chronic health problems.

Pathways for Home Health

To manage the patient with multiple diagnoses, the Home Health Services of Gottlieb Memorial Hospital in Melrose, Illinois, developed a generic clinical pathway that can be individualized to meet the patient's needs by completing blank spaces (Fig. 4–3). In the January 1994 issue of *Hospital Case Management,* the director of the program made the following suggestions about how to develop pathways for home health:

- Use phases of care rather than "weeks" of care.
- Limit duplication of charting entries.
- Provide accessibility to the pathway for all disciplines.
- Include provision of psychosocial and physical care during visits.
- Focus on case management activities common in home health such as assessment and education.
- Consider using a computer-based documentation system.

Clinical pathways for home health settings may also be developed according to specific medical diagnoses as in the acute care setting. After 2 years of development and testing of clinical pathways with the Center for Case Management of South Natick, Massachusetts, VNA First in Oak Park, Illinois, began using pathways for home care. Reimbursement changes in home health motivated VNA First to develop the pathways. As with hospital clinical pathways, patient outcomes and aspects or elements of care are listed.

VNA First also developed CoMap Tools, which are abbreviated pathways for comorbidities such as arthritis, chronic airway limitation, and hypertension. Many patients receiving home health care have multiple health problems that interrelate or affect the ability of the patient to meet the expected outcomes.

Time Frame: – a range of 1–5 x week for 8 weeks

GOTTLIEB MEMORIAL HOSPITAL
DEPARTMENT OF NURSING
CAREMAP

CASETYPE _____ Generic
PHYSICIAN _____
DRG _____
LOS _____

Day/Hour/Visit/Week

DATE: _____

	Week 1	Week 2	Week 3	Week 4
TEACHING/ ASSESSMENT	1. Follow generic plan for admission. 2. Assess knowledge of disease process. 3. Instruct on dressing changes, including aseptic technique. 4. Instruct on pain management. 5. Instruct on prosthetics/orthotics. 6. Instruct on emergency measures. 7. Assess knowledge of safety measures. 8. Assess psychosocial/emotional coping of patient and caregiver(s). 9. Instruct on nondurable equipment (Foley, ostomy, trach).	24. Assess knowledge of (medication). 25. Assess knowledge of (medication). 26. Assess knowledge of emergency measures. 27. Assess knowledge of diet. 28. Assess knowledge of prosthetics. 29. Instruct on skin care. 30. Assess ability to do dressing changes aseptically and safe disposal of wastes. 31. Instruct on safe body mechanics and positioning 32. Instruct on ROM. 33. Assess knowledge & effectiveness of pain management. 34. Assess status of disease process.	48. Assess knowledge of (medication). 49. Assess knowledge of and compliance with skin care regimen. 50. Assess utilization of safe body mechanics and positioning. 51. Assess ability to perform ROM exercises correctly and compliance with frequency. 52. Instruct on bladder program, i.e., bladder training, infection, retention, hygiene, 53. Instruct on bowel, i.e., continence, constipation and promotion of regularity. 54. Assess status of disease process.	67. Assess knowledge of (medication). 68. Assess knowledge of & compliance with bladder program. 69. Assess knowledge of & compliance with bowel program. 70. Assess knowledge of (medication). 71. Instruct on risk factors R/T diagnosis. 72. Instruct on relaxation technique
MEDICATIONS	10. Instruct on ____ 11. Instruct on ____	35. Instruct on (medication). 36. Assess compliance.	55. Instruct on (medication).	73. Instruct on (medication).
TREATMENTS	12. Weigh patient	37.	56.	74. Monthly Foley change if ordered.
TESTS	13. Draw labs as ordered/needed.	38.	57.	75.
ACTIVITY	14. Assess for proper use of DME's. 15. Homebound status must apply/ activity as tolerated	39.	58.	76. Instruct and/or assess for upgrade in activity level R/T diagnosis including sexual & job restrictions.
DIET	16. Initiate diet teaching, give appropriate information about ____ diet.	40. Follow thru with more in-depth diet teaching about ____ 41. Assess for compliance	59.	77.
OTHER DISCIPLINES	17. Contact other disciplines as determined R/T case type ____	42.	60. 61. Contact MD as needed for case management	78. 79.
NURSING DIAGNOSIS	18. Knowledge deficits ____ 19. ____ 20. ____	43. ____ 44. ____	62. ____ 63. ____	80. ____ 81. ____
PATIENT OUTCOMES/ DISCHARGE PLANNING	21. Knowledgeable regarding: ____ 22. ____ 23. ____	45. Can recognize and respond appropriately to an emergency. 46. Is independent in safe dressing changes. 47. Knowledgeable re: ____	64. ____ 65. Demonstrates knowledge of bowel and bladder regimens, 66. Uses good body mechanics and proper positioning.	82. Attainment of continence as able.

Continued on following page.

Figure 4–3   A generic clinical pathway used in a home health care agency. (Developed by Mary Noven, RN, and Debra K. Jansky, RN. Courtesy of Gottlieb Memorial Hospital, Melrose Park, Illinois.)

GOTTLIEB MEMORIAL HOSPITAL
DEPARTMENT OF NURSING
CAREMAP

CASETYPE _____ Generic
PHYSICIAN _____
DRG _____
LOS _____

Day/Hour/Visit/Week

Time Frame: – a range of
1 x week
for 8 weeks

DATE:	Week 5	Week 6	Week 7	Week 8

TEACHING/ ASSESSMENT	83. Assess knowledge of _____ (medication).
	84. Assess knowledge of risk factors R/T diagnosis.
	85. Assess knowledge and effectiveness of relaxation techniques.
	86. Assess knowledge of activity level and patient response.
	87. Instruct on community resources and assist patient to arrange for contact as needed.
	88. Instruct on how to obtain _____.
		101. Assess knowledge of _____ (medication).
		102. Assess knowledge of supply storage and procurement.
		103. Assess for discharge planning or recertification.
		104. _____
			116. Determine discharge based on knowledge of:
			  medications
			  diet
			  treatment
			  coping
			  pain management
			117. Assess status of disease process.
				125. Determine discharge based on knowledge of:
				  bladder program/
				  Foley care
				  bowel program
				  nondurable medical equipment
				  prosthetics/orthotics
				126. Complete client discharge information sheet with patient signature.
				127. Complete discharge summary.

MEDICATIONS	89. Instruct on _____ (medication). 90. Assess compliance	105.	118.	128.
TREATMENTS	91. Weigh patient		119.	129. Change Foley if ordered on monthly basis.
TESTS	92. Draw labs as ordered/indicated	106.	120.	
ACTIVITY	93. Homebound status	107.	121.	130. Independent with _____ 131.
DIET	94. Assess compliance.			
OTHER DISCIPLINES	95. Contact community resources as indicated.	108. Assess result of community resources contact. 109. Notify MD about initiation of discharge planning or recertification.		132. Notify MD of discharge status.
NURSING DIAGNOSIS	96. 97.	110. 111.		
PATIENT OUTCOMES/ DISCHARGE PLANNING	98. Can relate risk factors R/T diagnosis. 99. 100.	112. Pt./caregiver can follow up appropriately with community services. 113. Pt./caregiver will be able to obtain and store supplies correctly. 114. 115.	122. 123. 124.	133. Recertify due to _____ 134. 135.

CreMapHHS9

FIGURE 4–3 *Continued*

Pathways for Long-Term Care

Whether managed as an outpatient or in a nursing home, elderly patients have complex needs, making them unable to follow many of the clinical pathways used for younger patients. For this reason elderly patients are becoming a major focus of case management in a number of health care settings. For example, the case management program at Lutheran Healthcare Network in Meza, Arizona, focuses on people with chronic illnesses who are at high risk for using multiple acute care services. Case managers spend most of their efforts in educating patients to become more active in their own health care—a problem that is sometimes difficult to overcome when working with elderly patients (*Hospital Case Management,* March 1994).

To manage this population, Lutheran's clinical pathways typically extend beyond the walls of the hospital into the community. For example, Figure 4–4 illustrates a pathway for a patient with dementia being followed by a physician in the community. The timeline is based on visits rather than a specific period of time.

Although in its infancy, clinical pathway development is underway in some nursing home and chronic or extended care inpatient facilities (Fig. 4–5). One of the biggest obstacles to using pathways in these settings is the federal requirement for the facility to have a traditional interdisciplinary care plan for each patient. Although pathways could easily replace the current care plans, most state surveyors insist that the columnar format of patient problems, goals, interventions, and evaluation be used. As third-party payors and other accrediting bodies embrace the concept of pathways, these facilities may be able to abandon the traditional approach to care planning and use the more efficient and meaningful clinical pathway and case management system.

USE OF PATIENT PATHWAYS

Patient education is the central focus of health care in any setting. One of the primary uses for clinical pathways is patient education. At a glance the patient can see what events are expected and over what time frame they will occur. Many hospitals are in the process of adapting their interdisciplinary pathways to design patient versions (patient "itineraries") with less information and less jargon. This text has several samples of patient pathways in Appendix A.

To take the concept of patient pathways a step further, pictorial pathways and foreign-language pathways have been introduced in some settings (see Appendix C). Pictorial pathways are very simple and straightforward and are particularly useful for patients who are illiterate or unable to comprehend the written word. Figure 4–6 shows a sample used at Providence Hospital in Everett, Washington. When a patient comes to the hospital for preadmission testing for elective procedures, the pathway is explained, and each patient can take the pathway home for review. Physicians are generally supportive of this approach to patient education because the pathways are easy to understand.

The St. Vincent Infirmary Medical Center in Little Rock, Arkansas, presents its patient pathway to the patient in the physician's office before hospital admission. Standardized pathway brochures printed by the hospital are provided to the physicians' offices free of charge. Physicians have been very involved in developing the pathways at St. Vincent's Center. The case management staff at the hospital is also working with a Little Rock home health agency in pathway development for preadmission and postdischarge care (*Inside Case Management,* May 1994).

Some HMOs also use patient pathways. The Group Health Cooperative in Seattle, Washington, for instance, developed pictorial pathways balanced with

CONTINUING CARE PATHWAY
Dementia — Physician Office

Components	First 3 Visits	Follow-Up Visits Every 4 Months and as Needed
Assessment/Monitoring	• H&P focus on recent neuro changes: new lacunar infarct, EPSE from neuroleptic, Parkinson's features, cognitive changes • Care coordinator to complete assessment forms	———————————>
Consults	• SW • Consider PT, OT, rehab, psych, neuro geriatric assessment	• If cl. status changes, reconsider need for consults • Periodic communication w/other MD involved in care re:status & tx plan
Tests	• Dementia W/U if not already done (see protocol for W/U of memory loss/confusion) • Repeat bld work as needed	———————————>
Functional Rehab	• Assess for changes in function, cognition, behavior, gait, sleep, falls, wandering (helpful tools Folstein MM, Katz ADL) • Assess ability to continue driving • Assess for sensory loss—referral for eval. prn (audiology, etc.) • Exercise program to maintain conditioning	• Assess each visit for changes in function, cognitive & behavior ———————————>
Nutrition	• Baseline wt • Compare_ in last 4 mos–1 yr • Assess nutritional status & ability to chew, swallow & feed • Swallow eval. prn • Assess need for changes in consistency of diet—finger food, mech. diet, thick liquids, etc. (See nutrition guidelines) • Explore goals of long-term nutritional support (i.e., comfort vs. life prolonging methods) • Referral to outpt nutrition prn (696-7770)	• Assess each visit for changes in wt, nutritional status, appetite & ability to feed, chew & swallow • Reconsider need for nutritional consult prn ———————————>
Meds	• Review current & past meds including OTC • Assess for compliance to med regimen • Assess teaching needs re: meds, indication, dose, time, SE • Check for SE especially psychotropics-orthostatic_, anticholinergic, sedation, urinary retention, ↑ confusion, falls, EPSE, tardive dyskinesia	• Eval. effectiveness & ongoing use of meds ———————————> ———————————> • Ongoing instruction re: meds, indication, dose, time, S.E.
Treatment/Teaching	• Review course of dementia including common problems: behavior, falls, incont., sleep disturbances, wandering, etc. (see teaching material) • Provide education material on disease and community resources • Provide instruction for fall & safety precaution, B&B program, good skin care • Review advance directives & cl's goals of tx	• Re-evaluate ongoing teaching needs re: disease • Behavior management • Safety issues • Incontinence & toileting • Communication
Psychosocial	• Determine cl's ability to make decisions & need for surrogate decision maker • Assess for S&S of depression (helpful tool: depression scale) • Assess caregiver burden & social support—refer to support group and to Alzheimer's Association (708-933-2413) • Family mtg prn to address issues & goals • Refer cl/caregiver for counseling prn	• Ongoing assess of impact of condition on cl/caregiver ———————————> ———————————> ———————————>
Continuing Care Needs	• Assess current living situation & ability of caregiver to provide care • Assess cl safety at home especially for cl living alone • Consider referral for adult day care (696-7770), VNS (824-7720), for skilled needs or other in home support services, or NHP • Transition plan & paperwork provided to other sites of care • S.W. eval. prn to assist with decision & referrals to (696-7770 Senior I&R) • If no service in place, periodic f/u phone calls by care coordinator	• Reassess need for supportive services especially if cl status changes or support network changes • Periodic communication with other health professions providing care (VNA, day care) especially when cl status, meds or tx plan changes
	Signature: _____ Date: _____	Signature: _____ Date: _____

FIGURE 4-4 A clinical pathway for a patient with dementia being treated on an outpatient basis.

CONTINUING CARE PATHWAY
CVA - Skilled Nursing Facility
Short-Term Stay

Components	Admission-48 Hours	Week 1	Week 2	Ongoing	Discharge
Assessment/Monitoring	• Physician's H&P w/in 72hrs • M.D.S. w/in 7 days • Intradept. Assess (Nursing, Social Services Activity, Nutrition) • Vital signs as indic.	• Ongoing assessment & conf. of baseline data • Assess for causes in Δ from baseline • Ongoing assess. by therapist as to readiness for inpt rehab, home care or continued LTC	• Eval. by LGH rehab services to assess funct. potential (q wk) for poss. return to inpt rehab ————————>	• Assess cl/caregiver's ability to provide care for client going home ————————>	• Assess appropriateness of D/C plan • Update assess, forms & commun. status to new caregivers
Consults	• PT, OT, ST • Rehab physician prn • Nutrition prn (w/tube feeding, pressure sores or eating problems)	• Eval. for sensory losses & consult approp. services (i.e. audiology)	• Psych eval. prn for S&S depression		• Caregiver has arranged for follow-up w/MD p̄ D/C
Tests	• CBC, SMAC, U/A (w/in 72hrs), Mantoux Test • Protime if client on Coumadin————————>	• PT q̄ month or as indicated	• Swallow study prn to upgrade diet &/or D/C T,F		• Arrange for follow-up lab work prn
Functional/Rehab	• PT & OT • ST QD • OOB Bid • ROM/proper positioning • Safety & fall precaution prn • B&B program prn • Skin care prn • Assess & prevent complications from immobility	• Assess for Δs in functional status • Progress w/therapies based on cl endurance • Encourage independence for ADLs • ↑W/C tolerance to 3 hrs ————————>	————————> • Increase PT/OT to 3 hrs as tolerated (if returning to Rehab) • Assess cl/caregiver ability to meet rehab & self care needs ————————>	————————> • Weekly review to decide if cl progressing enough to cont. therapy ————————>	• Arrange for f/u therapies prn for client's going home
Nutrition	• Assess nutritional status, dietary needs & preferences • Baseline weights • Assess ability to chew & swallow • Nutrition consult prn	• Monitor po intake • Dietary Tech to review mthly for oral intake, supplements • Monitor tube feeding	• Supplement nutrition prn • Assess cl/caregiver knowledge of diet • Upgrade diet & wean T.F. per swallow study	• Monthly wts • Cl. tolerating adequate intake • Eval. need for G-tube prn if consistent w/goals • Dietary instruc. to cl/caregiver	• Cl/caregiver able to plan & provide proper diet • Communicate dietary needs & preferences to new caregivers.
Medication	• Anticoagulant therapy if indicated • Routine/PRN med as indicated • Assess ed. needs re: meds, indication dose, time, SE	————————> • Monitor response to meds • Instruct cl/caregiver re: meds	————————> ————————> ————————>	————————> • Cl. tolerating meds • Review approp. of current drug regimen every 30 days & prior to D/C	• Cl/caregiver can verbalize drug regimen • Written instruction provided

Continued on following page.

FIGURE 4–5 Example of a clinical pathway used in a nursing home. (Courtesy of Lutheran General Health System: The Pathway Project, Park Ridge, Illinois.)

CONTINUING CARE PATHWAY
CVA - Skilled Nursing Facility
Short-Term Stay Cont'd

Components	Admission-48 Hour	Week 1	Week 2	Ongoing	Discharge
Treatments/Teaching	• Assess cl/caregiver teaching needs re: condition, care, & tx plan • Review advance directives, code status & client's goals of tx.	• Instruct cl/caregiver re: condition, care & tx plan ——————>	——————>	• Review & update care plan quarterly ——————>	• Cl/caregiver verbalize/demonstrate knowledge of condition, care & tx plan
Spiritual	• Assess spiritual needs, i.e. values & preferences	• Offer options of spiritual support	——————>	——————>	• Spiritual needs are addressed
Psychosocial	• Assess impact of condition (i.e. depression, anxiety, loss) & coping in cl/caregiver • Consult psych. prn • Supportive counseling • Orient to new environment	• Involve in psychosocial &/or rec groups ——————> • Caregiver support PRN ——————> • Encourage visits & social outings	• Follow protocol for Depression if indicated ——————> ——————>	——————> ——————> ——————> ——————>	• Cl/caregiver demonstrate adequate coping • Referrals for ongoing counseling prn
Continuing Care Needs	• SW aware of cl/caregiver plans; rehab unit, home, long-term placement	• Review need for financial assistance prn • LGH rehab to periodic check status of client for possible return to inpt rehab • Assess caregiver's ability to care for client at home	• SW to arrange for LGH rehab/home care needs or provide emotional support for cont. NH placement • Home assessment by Therapies for clients going home	• Caregiver conference to discuss med tx, client goals, ongoing needs & D/C plan prn • SW follow-up for D/C plan, Rehab, Home, NH	• Cl. D/C w/approp. care, ie, home therapy, adult day care CORF • Referral back to LGH I&R if D/C w/no services

FIGURE 4–5 *Continued*

44

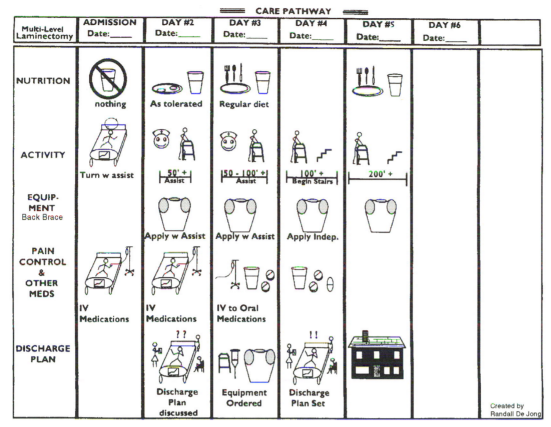

FIGURE 4–6   Example of a pictorial pathway used for patient education. (Courtesy of Providence General Medical Center, Everett, Washington. Created by Randall De Jong.)

text. Their patient pathways reduce the medical jargon to common language in a one-page format.

At St. Vincent's Hospital and Medical Center in Portland, Oregon, patient-oriented itineraries are provided to patients as part of an educational packet. At the top of the pathway, a note states the pathway is intended as a guideline only. Because Portland has a large Hispanic population, Spanish pathways have also been developed. Pictorial pathways may be used for other ethnic groups because of budgetary restraints (*Hospital Case Management,* August 1993). (See Appendix C of this book for samples of Spanish patient pathways.)

USE OF TOOLS TO MEASURE PATIENT OUTCOMES

The clinical pathways used by most health care facilities document whether or not the patient's outcomes were met. When the outcomes are not met, the case manager usually documents a reason that is included as part of variance analysis.

In an effort to be more comprehensive and customer oriented, some hospitals use a more extensive tool to measure outcomes as part of case management. For example, The Miriam Hospital in Providence, Rhode Island, developed outcome audit tools that are completed on the day of or the day before discharge. As shown in the example in Figure 4–7, all items require a "yes" or "no" answer. All negative answers must have a follow-up plan or referral. A major focus of the tool is on patient education to determine if the patient understands what the expectations are for him or her after hospital discharge.

THE MIRIAM HOSPITAL

CASE MANAGEMENT
AMI PATIENT OUTCOME AUDIT TOOL
DRG #122

ADDRESSOGRAPH

GUIDELINES:

Follow-up
Plan/referal

- Audit to be completed the day of discharge or the day before discharge.

- ALL items MUST have Yes or No answer.

- ALL negative responses REQUIRE follow-up plan and/or referral.

CHART DATA

Daily summaries/continued note/and/or flow sheet address:

a. Patient's breath sounds are clear or have returned to baseline.
                                        Yes _____   No _____

b. Patient has no peripheral edema or has returned to baseline.
                                        Yes _____   No _____

c. Cardiac rhythm is stable or pulse and BP are within normal limits
    for the patient.   Yes _____   No _____

RN INTERVIEW DATA

Interview the RN caregiver for the day. Ask the RN, "Can the patient
ambulate 30 feet without developing:"

a. Cardiac discomfort?   Yes _____   No _____

b. Dizziness?   Yes _____   No _____

c. S.O.B.?   Yes _____   No _____

PATIENT INTERVIEW DATA

Say to the patient: "Tell me, what would you do if you have cardiac
discomfort:"

a. Rest   Yes _____   No _____

b. Take NTG   Yes _____   No _____

c. Call EMS (911)   Yes _____   No _____

"Have all your questions and concerns been addressed while you have
been here?"   Yes _____   No _____

"What type of activity should you do when you go home?"

a. Gradually increase activity (walking) Yes _____   No _____

b. Rest when tired   Yes _____   No _____

FIGURE 4–7 Outcome audit tool to measure patient outcomes more specifically. (Used with permission of the Case Management Program, Miriam Hospital, Providence, Rhode Island.)

AMI Audit Tool
Page 2

Follow-up Plan/referal

"What activites shouldn't you do?"

a. Heavy lifting   Yes _____ No _____
b. Driving   Yes _____ No _____

"Do you have any of the following risk factors?
If yes, what is your plan?"

Smoking   Yes _____ No _____ Plan _____
High blood pressure Yes _____ No _____ Plan _____
High cholesterol   Yes _____ No _____ Plan _____
Obesity   Yes _____ No _____ Plan _____
Sedentary lifestyle Yes _____ No _____ Plan _____
Diabetes   Yes _____ No _____ Plan _____
Stress   Yes _____ No _____ Plan _____

Choose one medication that the patient will take home and ask:

a. What medication is for.   Yes _____ No _____
b. How often to take/day.   Yes _____ No _____
c. Time of day to take medication. Yes _____ No _____

"When is your appointment with your doctor?"
Patient gives date/time period.   Yes _____ No _____

"Have you considered attending a Cardiac
Rehabilitation Program?"   Yes _____ No _____

RN Signature _____

Date _____

7/92

Source: The Miriam Hospital, Providence, RI.

FIGURE 4–7 *Continued*   *Continued on following page.*

USE OF CLINICAL PATHWAYS AS PART OF THE DOCUMENTATION SYSTEM

As mentioned in Chapter 1, one of the potential problems with using pathways is that they are additional pieces of paper the nurse and other health team members are required to incorporate into daily practice. In some agencies the pathways are not a permanent part of the medical record, perhaps making them seem less important than other forms. More often than not, however, pathways are a part of the patient's permanent record.

Adding pieces to the record, however, may not be well accepted by some staff members. To overcome this objection, some hospitals have expanded their pathways to include patient care documentation in a charting-by-exception (CBE) type format. Figures 4–8 and 4–9 illustrate how two hospitals have incorporated documentation into the pathway. One of the concerns about this approach is that sometimes the documentation system is centered around nursing care. Other disciplines also must be able to document on the pathway if it is truly collaborative.

The use of CBE is also controversial. Some legal experts argue that CBE may be inadequate to protect the facility from liability. To answer this concern, additional space for narrative notes as needed can be provided on the back of the pathway. Each health care agency should consult legal experts if documentation is incorporated into its pathways.

USE OF PATHWAYS FOR DECISION MAKING

All clinical pathways used in hospitals do not necessarily track a patient along a preset timeline. For example, at Meriter Hospital in Madison, Wisconsin, obstetric staff wanted to reduce the number of inappropriate cesarean sections. A clinical pathway planning team designed four pathways, each an indicator that often leads to a cesarean section: vaginal birth after cesarean (previous cesarean), fetal distress, breech presentation, and dystocia. In the pathway for previous cesarean are indicators at pertinent points that direct the staff to use the other three pathways. The use of this type of decision-making tool has helped the hospital meet its overall goal of reducing its number of cesarean sections (*Critical Path Network,* May 1994).

▼ CHAPTER HIGHLIGHTS ▼

- Clinical pathways are being developed for many specialties within the hospital such as psychiatry and surgery.
- The timeline across the horizontal axis of the pathway may be in minutes, hours, days, or weeks.
- Less-specific timelines such as phases, intervals, or visits are also appropriate for pathways, depending on the health care setting.
- Clinical pathways are useful tools for patient education and staff orientation.
- Some clinical pathways track the patient across a continuum of care.
- Pathways may be used in any health care setting, including home health and long-term care.
- Patient pathways should be simple and without medical jargon; they may be pictorial or in a foreign language, depending on the patient's needs.
- Specific tools to measure patient outcomes are useful as a customer-oriented evaluation of patient care.

Daily Systems Assessment

WINCHESTER MEDICAL CENTER, INC.
Daily Systems Assessment

A ✔ is to be placed before appropriate criteria. – *Denotes comment on Nurses Progress Notes –N/A through section denotes not-applicable criteria

NEUROLOGICAL

LOC	ORIENTATION	SPEECH	PUPILS
__ Alert	__ Person	__ Clear	__ Equal
__ Lethargic	__ Place	__ Rambling	__ Unequal
__ Confused	__ Time	__ Dysphasic	__ Reactive
__ Arouses to pain		__ Aphasic	__ Pinpoint
__ Unresponsive		__ Slurred	__ Dilated

COMMENTS:_____

MUSCULOSKELETAL

__ Cast	__ Traction	__ Ice
__ Bil grips equal		__ Heat
__ Motion deficit	__ Sensation deficit	
__ RUE __ LUE	__ RUE	__ LUE
__ RLE __ LLE	__ RLE	__ LLE

COMMENTS:_____

CARDIOVASCULAR

PULSE	PERIPHERAL CHECK		EDEMA	SKIN	SKIN COLOR	TURGOR
__ Apical Rate	R L **Radial**	R L **Pedal**	__ None	__ Warm	__ No Abnormalities	__ Normal
__ Radial Rate	__ __ Strong	__ __ Strong	__ Peripheral	__ Dry	__ Pale	__ Abnormal
__ Regular	__ __ Weak	__ __ Weak	__ Sacral	__ Cool	__ Cyanotic	
__ Irregular	__ __ Thready	__ __ Thready	__ Other	__ Moist	__ Dusky	
__ Other	__ __ Bounding	__ __ Bounding		__ Clammy	__ Flushed	
	__ __ Absent	__ __ Absent		__ Dermal Ulcers	__ Jaundiced	
				__ Rash	__ Mottled	

COMMENTS:_____

RESPIRATORY

Respirations/Oxygenation		Breath Sounds
__ Regular	__ Chest Tube	R L
__ Shallow	__ Trach	__ __ Clear
__ Deep	__ O$_2$ __ L/Min	__ __ Rales
__ Labored	__ O$_2$ Device	__ __ Rhonchi
__ Cough		__ __ Wheeze
__ Sputum		__ __ Diminished
__ Audible Wheeze		__ __ Absent

COMMENTS:_____

GASTROINTESTINAL

GI Symptoms	Abdomen	Bowel Sounds
__ Difficulty Swallowing	__ Soft	__ Present
__ Nausea	__ Firm	__ Absent
__ Vomiting	__ Distended	__ Hyperactive
__ Bleeding	__ Tenderness	__ Hypoactive
__ Diarrhea	__ Ostomy	
__ Constipation	__ Tubes	

COMMENTS:_____

GENITOURINARY

__ Voiding s̄ difficulty	__ Retention	**Female**
__ Dysuria	__ Hematuria	__ Menses
__ Oliguria	__ Burning	__ Vaginal Discharge
__ Anuria	__ Dialysis	__ Unusual Bleeding
__ Nocturia	__ Foley	**Male**
__ Frequency	__ Tubes	__ Prostate Problems
__ Incontinence	__ Ostomy	__ Penile Discharge
	__ Irrigation	__ Unusual Bleeding

COMMENTS:_____

PSYCHO/SOCIAL

__ Appropriate	__ Apathetic
__ Inappropriate	__ Grieving
__ Uncooperative	__ Combative
__ Fearful/Anxious	__ Verbally Abusive
__ Flat	__ Physically Abusive
__ Defensive	__ Young/Old for Age
__ Hostile	
__ Non-Communicative	

COMMENTS:_____

POST-OP STATUS

Dressings	**Incision**	**Sutures/Staples**
__ Dry	__ Approximated	__ Intact
__ Drainage	__ Dry __ Hematoma	__ Removed
__ Reinforced	__ Red __ Swelling	
	__ Warm __ Drains	__ Steri Strips
	__ Tender __ Drainage	

COMMENTS:_____

EQUIPMENT

| __ Egg Crate |
| __ Specialty Mattress |
| __ Specialty Bed |
| Specify_____ |

ADDITIONAL COMMENTS:
_____
_____
_____
_____
_____

Date _____ Time _____ Signature _____

Source: Winchester Medical Center, Winchester, VA.   Rev 2/91   1/4/89

FIGURE 4–8 Example of an assessment flow sheet to accompany the clinical pathway. (Courtesy of Winchester Medical Center, Winchester, Virginia.)

ANNE ARUNDEL MEDICAL CENTER
ANNAPOLIS, MD. 21401
INTEGRATED RECORD-TOTAL KNEE REPLACEMENT

AGREES WITH PLAN OF CARE: _____

TEACHING PLAN: (KNOWLEDGE DEFICIT)   OUTCOMES

	INTERVENTIONS REVIEW:	PRE Initials/date	POST		CAN DEMONSTRATE/STATE	PRE Initials/date	POST
LEVEL	Breathing exercise (IS) goal			LEVEL	Use of Breathing exercise (IS)		
	View Video		■		Understanding of Video		■
	Use of equipment				Use of equipment		
	Explain Pain Scale (VAS)				Pain Scale 0-10 />5		
I	Reason for Blood Transfusion			I	Reason for Blood Transfusion		
	Activity restrictions				Activity restrictions		
	Reason for elastic stockings				Reason for elastic stockings		
	Review Pathway Progress	■			States Pathway Progress	■	
	Medications (Coumadin,_____)				Medications (Coumadin,_____)		
II	Do's and Dont's of Positioning			II	Do's and Dont's of Positioning		
	Review Pathway Progress	■			States Pathway Progress	■	
	Bowel Regimen				Bowel Regimen		
III	Instruct family: application of TEDS Knee Immobilizer	■		III	Application of TEDS Knee Immobilizer	■	
	Instruct proper use CPM controls				Proper use CPM controls		
	Review Pathway Progress				States Pathway Progress		
IV	Reason for prophylactic antibiotics before procedures			IV	Reason for prophylactic antibiotics before procedures		
	Review Pathway Progress	■			States Pathway Progress	■	
	Discharge Instructions	■			Discharge Instructions	■	
V	Notify Home Health of discharge when applicable	■		V	Notify Home Health of Discharge when applicable	■	
	Review Pathway Progress	■			States Pathway Progress	■	

DISCHARGE PLANNING: Impaired Home Health Management

	PRE	POST		PRE	POST
Soc. Work interview (Pt./Family)			H.H. Coord. meets patient/family	■	
Identify in-home care giver			Reviewed by Home Health	■	
Identify need for N.H. placement			Confirm Home services	■	
Level of care obtained	■		Other agency (Name, contact person, phone)		
Identification screen obtained	■				
N.H. Inquiries	■				
N.H. bed located	■				
Family completed N.H. paperwork	■		IDENTIFY EQUIPMENT NEEDS		ORDERED
Home Care Giver arranged	■		Hi Rise 3 in 1		
Discharge transportation arranged	■		Crutches		
Discharge plan completed			Walker		
			Other (specify):		
			Discharge Planning by: S.W., H.H. nurse or staff nurse		

SIGNATURE/TITLE:				

18-Mar-94

FIGURE 4–9   A different approach to including patient documentation into a clinical pathway. (Used with permission and developed by the Anne Arundel Medical Center, Annapolis, Maryland, staff and total knee clinical pathway team.)

ANNE ARUNDEL MEDICAL CENTER
ANNAPOLIS, MD. 21401
INTEGRATED RECORD-TOTAL KNEE REPLACEMENT

ACTIVITY: PHYSICAL MOBILITY   Key: ☐ Appropriate level   ▨ Needs qualifier See Progress Note

DATE:																Goals met/Initial/Date
Turn side to side X1-3																
Reinforce exercise X1-3																
Dangle as tolerated X1-3																
OOB chair X3																
Observe exercise X3																
Bed Mobility X3																
Ambulate to bathroom X1-3																
Ambulate in hall X2																
OOB chair X1																
Ambulate in hall X1																

INTERVENTIONS Shift	N	D	E	N	D	E	N	D	E	N	D	E	N	D	E	Goals met
IS Q 1h																
IS Q 2h when awake																
IS Q 4h when awake																
Reinforce Drsg. PRN																
TEDS off Q shift																
Knee immobilizer PRN																
Fall Prone Protocol																
CPM																
Prop heels/heel care																
Care level (Self)																
Care level (Partial)																
Care level (Complete)																
Hemovac DC'd																
PCA DC'd																
Dressing change																
IV to Saline lock or DC'd																
Saline lock DC'd																
Fleet enema PRN																
Discharge																

NUTRITIONAL ASSESSMENT/OUTCOMES

	Pre-op	Post-op	(*indicates RD intervention noted in progress notes)		
			Preadmission nutrition questionnaire completed		
			Nutritional risk assessed		
			Nutrition educational needs identified		
			Meal consumption goal met		
			Nutrition education/counselling completed		
			Discharge Rx:		
Signature/Title:					

18-Mar-94   FIGURE 4–9 *Continued*

- Some health care facilities are incorporating a documentation system as part of the clinical pathway; the format is typically charting by exception.
- Clinical pathways may be used as decision-making tools, especially in critical care settings such as labor and delivery.

5

Development of This Book's Clinical Pathways

This book uses the term *clinical pathway* to refer to what has also been called the *critical pathway, anticipated recovery path,* and many other terms. Clinical pathways are tools used to coordinate, plan, implement, monitor, and review patient care provided by the interdisciplinary health team. They serve as guides, rather than individualized care plans, and reflect the collaborative management of patient care.

The pathway samples in this book are intended for use in the hospital setting. Although clinical pathways have been initiated in other types of health care settings such as home care and rehabilitation, they are not used as universally in those settings as in hospitals. The focus of this book's clinical pathways in Part II is on adult medical-surgical health problems, including medical diagnoses and procedures. Some of the samples in the book are intended for use in the critical care setting (see Part III). Chapter 4 includes examples of pathways used in health care agencies other than hospitals.

CHARACTERISTICS OF THE CLINICAL PATHWAYS

Development of Clinical Pathways

As described in the previous chapters, there are a number of ways to conceptualize and develop clinical pathways. The authors approached pathway development by first reviewing the literature describing the usual management of hospitalized patients admitted with each medical diagnosis or procedure. The focus of the literature search was on the uncomplicated, "typical case" that was predictable and followed a pattern.

The authors then reviewed medical records from several hospitals to determine how closely actual practice followed the literature descriptions. They then reviewed and analyzed clinical pathways from hospitals across the United States that were willing to share their ideas. Finally, the authors synthesized all available information to present samples that can be modified to meet individual hospital and health care team preferences. All clinical pathways were reviewed by members of the health care team before publication (see reviewer list at the beginning of the book).

Description of Clinical Pathways

The clinical pathways in this book are comprehensive, incorporating as much useful information as possible. The pathways were selected by their frequency of occurrence and how easily they would fit a pattern. They are clinically oriented and designed as a permanent part of the medical record.

Bower (1994) states that 80% of all hospital admissions have medical diagnoses with fairly predictable patterns. These patients are in the "high-volume" category. The remaining 20% are in the "high-risk" or "high-cost" categories, most likely as a result of medical complications, multiple health problems, or the complex nature of the diagnoses. This book includes diagnoses primarily from the high-volume group, although some high-volume diagnoses are also high cost or high risk.

COMPONENTS OF THE CLINICAL PATHWAYS

The information at the top of each pathway includes the name of the health problem (medical diagnosis or procedure) with its associated international diagnostic code, 9th edition (ICD-9 code). In most cases the ICD-9 code is more specific than the DRG identification. The expected hospital length-of-stay (ELOS) is also listed at the top of the pathway as a guide. The ELOS for each of the book's pathways is based on the literature, actual practice, and the Health Care Financing Administration (HCFA). HCFA is the federal agency that sets the guidelines for reimbursement by Medicare in the United States.

Each hospital determines what its ELOS for each clinical pathway should be. The goal is to discharge the patient as soon as possible by using coordinated discharge planning, including patient and family education.

Nursing Diagnoses/Collaborative Problems

Some health care agencies do not incorporate nursing diagnoses into their pathways. Their argument against doing so is that the pathway is an interdisciplinary, rather than a nursing, tool. Others argue that all members of the health care team can comprehend most of the nursing diagnoses and find them useful in their practice. For example, *impaired verbal communication* is appropriate terminology for the speech/language pathologist. *Pain* is the term for a problem that all health team members can treat within their areas of clinical expertise and scope of practice.

Another argument in favor of including nursing diagnoses is that most case managers are nurses and therefore can use nursing diagnoses in their practice as a manager of patient care. Although there is no one answer to this controversy, the authors of this book chose to include nursing diagnoses and collaborative problems to focus primarily on actual concerns associated with each medical diagnosis or procedure.

The first section of the pathway lists the nursing diagnoses and collaborative problems commonly associated with the specified health problem. Because the clinical pathways that represent high-volume problems are somewhat predictable based on health care literature and practice, nursing diagnoses and collaborative problems are also predictable. That is, given a certain medical diagnosis, most patients experiencing that diagnosis will have certain nursing diagnoses or collaborative problems.

Some experts in nursing diagnosis do not agree that nursing diagnoses can be predictable. They believe that each patient is an individual and therefore no two patients experiencing the same health problem would have the same nursing diagnoses. This rather narrow view of nursing diagnosis is being challenged around the world (NANDA Conference, 1994).

In reality, all patients with a common health problem such as cerebrovascular accident (CVA) have *some* nursing diagnoses or collaborative problems in common. For example, hospitalized patients experiencing a CVA typically have the following nursing diagnosis labels: "Impaired physical mobility, Self-care deficit, and Altered (cerebral) tissue perfusion." Patients with a myocardial infarction experience "Decreased cardiac output and Activity intolerance."

The etiologies for these diagnostic labels are usually added to make a two-part statement for a complete nursing diagnosis (e.g., "Impaired physical mobility related to weakness of the right side"). However, for the clinical pathways in this book, the etiologies for actual problems or risk factors for high-risk problems are not specified. The authors chose this approach because the etiologies or risk factors are usually very specific to each patient; the pathway is a guide for *all* patients with a given medical diagnosis or procedure.

For each clinical pathway, a list of common nursing diagnoses and collaborative problems is located at the top of the pathway. The nursing diagnoses come from those labels included in the most recent North American Nursing Diagnosis Association (NANDA, 1994) list (Appendix B). The collaborative problems are similar to those developed by Carpenito (1993). Collaborative problems are disease or treatment complications the nurse monitors, prevents, assesses, or reports to the physician for medical intervention. For example, hypoglycemia is a complication (collaborative problem) that can occur in a diabetic patient. The collaborative problem may be stated as "Potential for hypoglycemia" or "PC (potential complication): hypoglycemia."

Expected Outcomes

For each nursing diagnosis or collaborative problem, at least one expected patient outcome is listed. This outcome states what the *patient* is expected to accomplish by the hospital discharge date. To minimize liability, the statement "the patient is expected to . . ." is used instead of the traditional "the patient will . . .."

The discharge outcome may not be the ultimate long-term goal for the patient. For instance, a patient who had a total hip replacement may be able to bear weight partially using a walker while walking from the room into the hall by the hospital discharge date. The long-term goal in another 6 to 8 weeks after intensive rehabilitation, however, might be that the patient can walk independently with a cane for 100 feet using full weight bearing. Some hospitals include both the discharge outcomes and the outcomes for the entire continuum of care. Other health care agencies specify outcomes for each phase of care.

The column adjacent to the list of expected outcomes at the top of the pathway is labeled "Met/Not Met." The case manager fills in this column and initials each outcome at the time of the patient's discharge. Ideally, all listed patient outcomes should be met by discharge. If not, the case manager indicates that the outcome was not met and documents an explanation in the next column labeled "Reason." The information in this column is a variance—a deviation from the clinical pathway—that is recorded and analyzed at a later time. Table 5–1 provides an example of the expected outcome portion of a clinical pathway for total hip replacement.

Timeline

Across the top of the actual pathway is a timeline for sequencing interventions for patient care. In a noncritical care hospital unit the time intervals are usually day by day. A column for preadmission and preoperative interventions is also included for elective surgical procedures.

In a critical care unit such as coronary care, emergency department, or operating suite, the timeline is often hour by hour, at least for the first few hours after admission. Once the patient is stabilized, the timeline may be extended to daily intervals, depending on the stay in the unit.

Table 5–1   **Example of Documenting Expected Outcomes**

Clinical Pathway for Total Hip Replacement
ICD-9 Code **715.35**   ELOS **6 days**

Nursing Diagnosis/ Collaborative Problem	Expected Outcome (The patient is expected to . . .)	Met/Not Met	Reason
Pain	State that pain is relieved after appropriate interventions		
Potential for hip dislocation	Not experience dislocation of the operative hip		
Potential for postoperative complications (hemorrhage, infection, thromboembolitic complications)	Have Hgb & Hct WNL, stable VS, WBC WNL, and no S/S of DVT, PE, or other thromboembolitic complications		
Impaired physical mobility	Walk from room into hall using a walker with supervision; not experience complications of immobility		

Recognizing the extreme variability among practitioners and the specificity of acute, complex health problems in critical care settings, this book's pathways do not include timeline intervals of less than a day-to-day sequencing. Users of these pathways can modify them, however, for their particular agencies.

The pathways in this book also do not specify a timeline interval for postdischarge care, although discharge planning is included as an aspect of care. Postdischarge care to home or other health care agency is specific to the individual setting in each community. Therefore for the book's generic pathways this information was not included. Some hospitals have incorporated postdischarge care as part of their clinical pathways in collaboration with specific community agencies.

Aspects of Patient Care

The pathway itself is divided into important aspects of care (down the vertical axis) across the timeline (horizontal axis). The specific aspects of patient care are typically selected by each hospital as part of pathway development. The samples in this book include 11 aspects of care:

- Assessment
- Teaching
- Consults
- Laboratory (lab) tests
- Other tests
- Medications (meds)
- Treatments/interventions
- Nutrition
- Lines/tubes/monitors
- Mobility/self-care
- Discharge planning

Assessment

The assessment section of the clinical pathway focuses on the physical and psychosocial assessments that the nurse performs for the patient with the specified

Teaching-Learning Record for Insulin Self-Administration			
Steps	Taught/Demonstrated (Initial)	Date	Return Demonstration (Initial)
1. Selects correct insulin type.			
2. Selects correct syringe.			
3. Cleans top of vial.			
4. Draws up correct insulin amount(s).			
5. Selects appropriate site for injection.			
6. Cleans skin with alcohol wipe.			
7. Uses 90-degree angle when injecting insulin.			

FIGURE 5–1 Example of a patient teaching record. (From Ignatavicius, D., Workman, L., & Mishler, M. (1995). *Medical-surgical nursing. A nursing process approach*, 2nd ed. Philadelphia: W.B. Saunders.

health problem. For example, the nurse assesses for signs and symptoms of hip dislocation (pain, shortening, and rotation of the affected limb) for the patient who had total hip replacement. The nurse continues this assessment and monitoring during the entire hospital stay as indicated across the 5-day hospital stay (see clinical pathway on total hip replacement).

In this book's pathways general systems assessment is also listed to reflect the need for nurses and other health care professionals to perform routine assessments required for all patients, regardless of diagnosis or procedure.

Teaching

The teaching aspect of care includes the ongoing education that the patient and family need for both the hospital stay and home or alternative care setting. This aspect focuses on interdisciplinary patient education. For example, the patient who has a total hip replacement needs teaching about leg exercises, positioning, and pain management. The patient with congestive heart failure needs teaching about a sodium-restricted diet.

The clinical pathways in this book list the family under "Teaching." The term *family* includes relatives, significant others, and other caregivers who are or will be responsible for patient care.

The teaching components in this segment of the pathway often reflect the specified nursing diagnoses or collaborative problems. For instance, teaching about a sodium-restricted diet is an intervention for the nursing diagnosis label of "Fluid volume excess." In many hospitals a supplementary teaching record such as the one shown in Figure 5–1, elaborates on the specific content to be taught and requires the person(s) providing the teaching to document the teaching-learning process.

Consults

The consults section lists members of the interdisciplinary team who are routinely needed to help the patient meet the expected outcomes. For the patient with a total hip replacement, those members typically include, but are not limited to, a physical therapist and a social worker.

Laboratory Tests

The laboratory tests required to monitor the patient before and during the hospital stay are included. Specific preadmission tests are not consistently listed in this book's pathways because they are typically determined by each hospital. The results of the laboratory tests help the interdisciplinary team decide if additional interventions are necessary. Some postoperative total hip replacement patients, for example, need a blood transfusion when the hemoglobin and hematocrit values markedly decrease from their preoperative levels.

Other Tests

The other diagnostic tests are listed in this section. An x-ray of the surgical hip is typically done several days after a total hip replacement. Including the hip x-ray in this segment of the pathway reminds the health team in advance that the x-ray examination must be scheduled and arrangement for transportation to the x-ray department must be made.

Medications

The medications section lists the typical medications prescribed for the patient. For example, the postoperative patient with a total hip replacement often uses a Patient-controlled analgesia (PCA) pump with either morphine or meperidine (Demerol) for the first 48 hours after surgery for pain control. Then an oral opioid analgesic such as oxycodone and acetaminophen (Tylox) is prescribed. An intravenous cephalosporin is administered during the first 24 hours, and warfarin (Coumadin), heparin, or enoxaparin (Lovenox) is prescribed over the course of the hospital stay. The patient is usually discharged with a physician's order for warfarin therapy to prevent thromboembolitic complications postoperatively.

Treatments/Interventions

The treatments portion of this aspect of patient care focuses on physician-directed treatments such as dressing changes, tube irrigations, and intermittent catheterizations. Medications are not included in this aspect of care because they are listed in the section entitled "Meds."

Interventions are those actions that do not usually require a physician's order. These interventions may be facility protocols, predetermined standards of care, or independent nursing actions. For example, a patient with a Foley catheter requires catheter care at least daily, which typically means that the perineal area is cleansed with soap and water, rinsed well, and patted dry. The Foley catheter should be secured by a leg strap to the thigh (female) or tape to the abdomen (male). Foley catheter care is a typical nursing standard of care. Therefore the clinical path may state "Foley catheter care according to unit standard" if unit standards are used.

In addition to written standards, the nurse often performs independent nursing actions such as checking the patient's heels every 8 hours for tenderness or skin breakdown. These interventions are usually those actions that address the specified nursing diagnoses at the top of the pathway. Monitoring a patient's heels is an intervention for the nursing diagnosis label of Impaired physical mobility.

Nutrition

The nutrition aspect of care includes the special nutritional needs of the patient and any dietary restrictions. Nutritional interventions are separated from the Treatments/Interventions section to illustrate the importance of nutritional assessment and interventions for patients with actual health problems or as part of a plan to help prevent health problems.

Lines/Tubes/Monitors

This aspect of patient care specifies the infusion therapy routes, monitors (e.g., cardiac monitors), and tubes such as drains and catheters that the patient has in place. For infusion therapy most clinical pathways list the usual infusion solutions that are administered in a particular health care agency. This information also helps the nurse know when to expect discontinuation of the lines, monitors, or tubes.

Mobility/Self-Care

Mobility and self-care needs are specified for each patient. For example, the patient who had a total hip replacement with a cemented prosthesis is permitted to bear weight to tolerance on the affected leg using a walker for ambulation. While in bed, the patient may turn to the unaffected side while keeping the legs abducted with one or more pillows.

Information in this segment of the clinical pathway usually is geared to physical and occupational therapists, but nurses and other health care providers need to follow and reinforce the information with the patient.

Discharge Planning

In the section entitled "Discharge Planning," the plans for patient discharge are listed, including needs and resources. For instance, the patient having a total hip replacement requires rehabilitation in a rehabilitation center or skilled nursing facility for 6 to 8 weeks. The social worker or other discharge planner makes the arrangements for placement and transfer to the postdischarge facility. The interdisciplinary team involves the patient, family, and significant others in the discharge planning process.

The information in the discharge planning section ties in with the expected outcomes. For example, if outcomes in the hospital have not been met, a plan to meet the outcomes after discharge must be developed.

▼ CHAPTER HIGHLIGHTS ▼

- Clinical pathways are tools used to coordinate, plan, implement, monitor, and review patient care that is provided by the interdisciplinary health team.
- Clinical pathways may include a list of nursing diagnoses or collaborative problems as this book does.
- Expected patient outcomes are a very important part of the clinical pathway.
- The timeline on the pathways is often daily but may be hourly for critical care settings.
- The clinical pathway consists of identified aspects of care that are agency specific; this book's pathways identify 11 aspects of care.

▼ ▼ ▼ ▼ ▼ ▼ ▼ ▼ ▼ ▼ ▼

Selected Bibliography

Acord-Szczesny, J. (1994, May). Computer tracking of critical path variations. *Inside Case Management,* pp. 1–3.

Bower, K. (1992). *Case management by nurses.* Kansas City: American Nurses Publishing.

Bower, K. (1994). Presentation at the North American Diagnosis Association Conference, March, 1994.

Coffey, R.J., Richards, J.S., Remmert, C.S., et al. (1992). An introduction to critical paths. *Quality Management in Health Care, 1*(1), 45–54.

Cohen, E.L. (1991). Nursing case management: Does it pay? *Journal of Nursing Administration, 21*(4), 20–25.

Cohen, E.L., & Cesta, T.G. (1993). *Nursing case management: From concept to evaluation.* St. Louis: Mosby–Year Book.

Critical Path Network (1993, May). Generic pathways can lead to individualized documentation, pp. 89–90.

Critical Path Network (1994, April). Integrated clinical pathway documentation; It works! pp. 63–64.

Critical Path Network (1994, May). Better critical pathway compliance leads to fewer C-sections, pp. 81–82.

Crummer, M.B., & Carter, V. (1993). Critical pathways—the pivotal tool. *Journal of Cardiovascular Nursing, 7*(4), 30–37.

Gosfield, A. (1994, August). Eight attributes of good clinical practice guidelines. *Inside Case Management,* pp. 1–2.

Grau, L. (1992). Case management and the nurse. *Geriatric Nursing, 13*(6), 372–375.

Graybeal, K.B., Gheen, M., & McKenna, B. (1993). Clinical pathway development: The Overlake model. *Nursing Management, 24*(4), 42–45.

Gruliano, K.K., & Porrer, C.E. (1991). Nursing case management: Critical paths to desirable outcomes. *Nursing Management, 22*(3), 52–55.

Guthrie, S. (1994, May). Clinical pathways become patient pathways. *Inside Case Management,* pp. 3–4.

Hampton, D.C. (1993). Implementing a managed care framework through care maps. *Journal of Nursing Administration, 23*(5), 21–27.

Heacock, D., & Brobst, R. (1994, July). A multidisciplinary approach to critical path development. *Journal of Nursing Care Quality,* pp. 38–41.

Hicks, L., Stallmeyer, J., & Coleman, J. (1992, July-August). Nursing challenges in managed care. *Nursing Economics,* pp. 165–276.

Hofman, P.A. (1993, June). Critical path method: An important tool for coordinating clinical care. *Journal of Quality Improvement,* pp. 235–246.

Hospital Case Management (1993, February). Clinical progression maps, pp. 27–30.

Hospital Case Management (1993, March). Why Alliant and Toronto hospitals are reassessing hundreds of paths, pp. 41–45.

Hospital Case Management (1993, August). Keep focus on the big picture when tackling variance analysis, pp. 150–152.

Hospital Case Management (1993, August). Pictorial pathways offer itineraries of hospital experience for patients, pp. 137–142.

Hospital Case Management (1993, September). CM credentials questioned as experts debate who's best qualified for the job, pp. 153–157.

Hospital Case Management (1993, October). The next wave of hospital case management: Mapping out psychiatric diagnoses on paths, pp. 173–177.

Hospital Case Management (1994, January). Rehab programs turn to case management models to improve quality, reduce LOS, pp. 1–6.

Hospital Case Management (1994, February). Paths are no substitution for good documentation, pp. 33–34.

Hospital Case Management (1994, March). Hospitals use case management to help elderly navigate the health care continuum, pp. 37–42.

Hospital Case Management (1994, June). 1995 continuum-of-care standards suited to case management, pp. 95–96, 101.

Hospital Case Management (1994, July). Hospitals use practice data to garner physician support, pp. 121–124.

Hospital Case Management (1994, November). Simple communication tips can save hours of anxiety, p. 187.

Joseph, E.D. (1994, September). The statistical imperative. *Inside Case Management,* p. 6.

Keatley, M.A. (1994, September). Managing care through outcomes analysis. *Inside Case Management,* p. 7.

Lucas, C. (1994, April). Mastering change: A case manager's perspective. *Inside Case Management,* pp. 1–3.

Mann, V.A. (1993). Clinical case management: A service line approach. *Nursing Management, 23*(9), 48–50.

Merry, M.D. (1994, May). The death of a paradigm. *Inside Case Management,* p. 8.

Miller, T.I. (1994, May). Taking the numb out of numbers for case managers. *Inside Case Management,* pp. 6–7.

Milne, C., & Romar, D. (1994, April). Choosing the right data base. *Inside Case Management,* pp. 7–8.

Mosher, C., Cronk, P., Kidd, A., et al. (1992). Upgrading practice with critical pathways. *American Journal of Nursing, 92*(1), 41–44.

Mullahy, C. (1992). Case managers and physicians: Working associates, not adversaries. *Case Manager, 3*(2), 62–68.

Nelson, M.S. (1993). Critical pathways in the emergency department. *Journal of Emergency Nursing, 19*(2), 110–114.

Sinnen, M.T., & Schifalacqua, M. (1991). Coordinated care in a community hospital. *Nursing Management, 22*(3), 38–42.

St. Luke's Episcopal Hospital (1994, May). Focusing on outcomes. *RN,* pp. 57–60.

Wagie, T., & Krausher, V. (1994, April). Nine steps to choosing case types variances. *Inside Case Management,* pp. 3–4.

Wall, D.K., & Proyect, M.M. (1994, November). Pitching pathways: Selling upper management on the value of critical pathway development, pp. 1–2.

Weilitz, P.B., & Potter, P.A. (1993). A managed care system: Financial and clinical evaluation. *Journal of Nursing Administration, 23*(11), 51–57.

Weinman, H. (1994, June). Case management: One physician's view. *Inside Case Management,* pp. 5–6.

Williams, R. (1992). Nursing case management: Working with the community. *Nursing Management, 23*(12), 33–34.

Wood, R.G., Bailey, N.O., & Tilkemeter, D. (1992). Managed care: The missing link in quality improvement. *Journal of Nursing Care Quality, 6*(4), 55–65.

Zander, K. (1991). Care maps: The core of cost/quality care. *New Definition, 6*(3), 1–3.

Zander, K. (1992). Quantifying, managing, and improving quality. Part III: Using variance concurrently. *New Definition, 7*(4), 1–4.

Zander, K., & McGill, R. (1994, August). Critical and anticipated recovery paths: Only the beginning. *Nursing Management,* pp. 34–40.

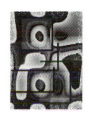

Part II

Clinical Pathways for Medical-Surgical Patients

Unit

I

Problems of Oxygenation/ Respiratory Health Problems

▼ ▼ ▼

Clinical Pathway for Laryngectomy

ICD-9 Code **161.9**   ELOS **7 days**

Nursing Diagnosis/Collaborative Problem	Expected Outcome (The Patient Is Expected to...)	Met/Not Met	Reason	Date/Initials
Ineffective airway clearance and ineffective breathing pattern	Maintain a patent airway and effective breathing pattern			
Pain	State pain is relieved or controlled with PO medication			
Impaired verbal communication	Communicate with family and visitors using appropriate assistance devices			
Altered nutritional status	Have adequate nutritional intake orally or through a feeding tube			

Aspect of Care	Date___ Pre-admission/Pre-op	Date___ Day 1 (ICU) (DOS)	Date___ Day 2 (ICU) (POD #1)	Date___ Day 3 (POD #2)	Date___ Day 4 (POD #3)	Date___ Day 5 (POD #4)	Date___ Day 6 (POD #5)	Date___ Day 7 (POD #6)
Assessment	Systems assessment with attention to • Oral cavity • Voice quality • Nutritional and respiratory status; Monitor for dysphagia, dyspnea, pain; Pre-op check list; Psychosocial assessment	*PACU:* Systems and pain assessment; VS q 15 min x 4, then q 30 min x 2; Check dressing for drainage q 1 h; Ensure all drains/tubes patent	System and pain assessment; VS q 2 h; Check dressing for bleeding; Ensure all drains/tubes patent; Monitor for complications • Hemorrhage • Respiratory distress	Systems and pain assessment; VS q 4 h; Check incision for bleeding, infection; Ensure all drains/tubes patent; Monitor for complications • Hemorrhage	Same as Day 3	Same as Day 4	Same as Day 5; VS q 8 h	Same as Day 6

Check ventilator settings *Post-op ICU:* Systems and pain assessment VS q 1 h Check ventilator settings Check dressing for drainage q 1 h × 8 Ensure all drains/tubes patent Monitor for complications • Hemorrhage • Respiratory distress	• Respiratory distress • Atelectasis • Pneumonia Monitor for anxiety, body image disturbance						
Teaching Orient to hospital and unit Reinforce information about surgery • Incision location • Tubes and drains • Post-op care – ICU – TCDB – Leg exercise *PACU:* Pain management *Post-op:* Reinforce information from pre-op teaching	Reinforce information about communication system	Self-suctioning techniques Instruct to cover trach when coughing Principles of speech therapy: esophageal speech Prepare for transfer out of ICU	Same as Day 3 Coping with body image issues	Home care • Bathing • Trach/stoma care • Humidification • Covering stoma for shower, shave, hair cuts	Care of feeding tube (if applicable) or begin swallowing and eating program per protocol	Continue feeding program Exercise program and importance of avoiding fatigue

Continued

Clinical Pathway for Laryngectomy *Continued*

Aspect of Care (Cont'd)	Date ___ Pre-admission/ Pre-op	Date ___ Day 1 (ICU) (DOS)	Date ___ Day 2 (ICU) (POD #1)	Date ___ Day 3 (POD #2)	Date ___ Day 4 (POD #3)	Date ___ Day 5 (POD #4)	Date ___ Day 6 (POD #5)	Date ___ Day 7 (POD #6)
Teaching (Cont'd)	– Pain management – Communication – Neck exercises – Tube feedings Encourage to verbalize fears and ask questions Importance of meticulous oral hygiene Have person who has had laryngectomy visit Prepare for loss of other abilities: sense of smell, sipping, using straw (total laryngectomy) Involve family in care of patient as appropriate Review plan of care/clinical pathway with patient and family					Instruct to notify MD of signs of respiratory infection, esophagitis, esophageal stenosis		

	Day 1	Day 2	Day 3	Day 4	Day 5	Day 6	Day 7
Consults	Medical clearance for surgery Social worker *Post-op:* Dietician Respiratory therapy	Rehab services • PT, OT • Speech	N/A	N/A	N/A	N/A	N/A
Lab Tests	CBC with diff, SMA-20, Cr, INR(PT)/APTT Type and screen U/A *Post-op:* Hgb and Hct ABGs	N/A ABGs before ventilator D/C'd	SMA-6(60) Hgb and Hct	SMA-6(60) Hgb and Hct	N/A	N/A	N/A
Other Tests	Chest, skull, sinus, neck x-rays CT neck, larynx MRI larynx, neck, brain, bone, liver ECG	N/A	Chest x-ray	N/A	N/A	N/A	N/A
Meds	IV broad-spectrum antibiotics before surgery *PACU:* Analgesics via PCA pump or IM *Post-op:* Analgesia via PCA pump or IM IV antibiotics x 7 days	Same as Day 1	D/C PCA pump Analgesia via feeding tube or IM (opioid or nonopioid) Continue broad-spectrum antibiotics	Analgesia via feeding tube D/C opioid analgesia Continue antibiotics	Same as Day 4	Same as Day 5	Same as Day 6

Continued

Clinical Pathway for Laryngectomy Continued

Aspect of Care (Cont'd)	Date___ Pre-admission/ Pre-op	Date___ Day 1 (ICU) (DOS)	Date___ Day 2 (ICU) (POD #1)	Date___ Day 3 (POD #2)	Date___ Day 4 (POD #3)	Date___ Day 5 (POD #4)	Date___ Day 6 (POD #5)	Date___ Day 7 (POD #6)
Treatments/ Interventions	Calorie count Wt	*PACU:* Trach care Suction PRN Semi-Fowler's or Fowler's position Strict I & O *Post-op:* Trach care Suction PRN Measure drainage from JP/Hemovac q 8 h Semi-Fowler's or Fowler's position Oral care QID Thigh-high antiembolism stockings and SCDs Support back, head, and neck	Trach care Suction PRN Semi-Fowler's or Fowler's position Measure JP/ Hemovac q 8 h Oral care QID Thigh-high antiembolism stockings and SCDs Support back, head, and neck Begin neck exercises Incentive spirometer q 1–2 h W/A Wt	Same as Day 2 except • D/C SCDs	Trach care Suction PRN Semi-Fowler's or Fowler's position Oral care QID Thigh-high antiembolism stockings Support back, head, and neck; neck exercises Incentive spirometer q 4 h W/A Wt I & O	Laryngeal tube care Suction PRN Elevate HOB 30° Oral care QID Thigh-high antiembolism stockings Incentive spirometer QID Neck exercises BID Wt I & O	Same as Day 5	Same as Day 6

Nutrition	NPO after midnight	NPO until bowel sounds present, then begin tube feeding per protocol TPN if malnourished	Tube feeding per protocol or TPN	Same as Day 2	Same as Day 3	Tube feedings Swallow evaluation (hemilaryngectomy)	Tube feedings Swallow evaluation (total) Progress diet per protocol based on swallowing evaluation	Same as Day 6
Lines/Tubes/Monitors	N/A	Continuous IV fluids Trach Hemovac/JP drain Nasogastric, gastrostomy or jejunostomy tube Foley cath Ventilator Cardiac monitor	D/C ventilator D/C Foley Humidification via trach collar IV fluids 50 mL/h Feeding tube Cardiac monitor	Saline loc if tolerates tube feedings D/C Hemovac/JP	Saline loc	Same as Day 4 D/C trach (hemilaryngectomy)	Saline loc Trach (if total)	D/C Saline loc Change trach tube to laryngectomy tube
Mobility/Self-Care	Activity as tolerated	Bed rest TCDB q 2 h ROM q 4 h w/a Prevent complications of immobility	OOB to chair BID ROM q 4 h TCDB q 2 h Prevent complications of immobility	OOB to chair TID or as tolerated Ambulate in room	OOB and ambulate in hall as tolerated	Same as Day 4	Same as Day 5	Same as Day 6

Continued

Clinical Pathway for Laryngectomy Continued

Aspect of Care (Cont'd)	Date___ Pre-admission/ Pre-op	Date___ Day 1 (ICU) (DOS)	Date___ Day 2 (ICU) (POD #1)	Date___ Day 3 (POD #2)	Date___ Day 4 (POD #3)	Date___ Day 5 (POD #4)	Date___ Day 6 (POD #5)	Date___ Day 7 (POD #6)
Discharge Planning	N/A	Assess need for social services, financial status, health insurance and coverage, home environment, need for placement and family support	Same as Day 1 Question family about area to clean laryngeal tube	Assess ability to perform ADLs, home environment, and need for assistive/ adaptive devices	Refer to home health Instruct on need to humidify home Instruct to obtain Medi-Alert bracelet	Ensure home health and rehab visits arranged Refer to International Association of Laryngectomies and American Cancer Society	Ensure communication system understood by all home caregivers	Arrange for follow-up visit with MD

Notes

Clinical Pathway for Pneumonia

ICD-9 Code 090   ELOS 5 days

Nursing Diagnosis/ Collaborative Problem	Expected Outcome (The Patient Is Expected to...)	Met/ Not Met	Reason	Date/ Initials
Impaired gas exchange	Demonstrate effective use of pursed lip and diaphragmatic breathing and controlled coughing techniques			
Ineffective breathing pattern	Demonstrate effective use of pursed lip and diaphragmatic breathing and controlled coughing techniques			
Ineffective airway clearance	Maintain clear and patent airway through coughing and deep breathing			
Fatigue	Return to usual activity level			

Aspect of Care	Date___ Day 1	Date___ Day 2	Date___ Day 3	Date___ Day 4	Date___ Day 5
Assessment	Systems assessment q shift with focus on respiratory • Rate, rhythm, depth • Chest expansion • Color, tenacity, and amt of sputum • Adventitious breath sounds • Accessory muscle utilization VS q 4 h	Same as Day 1	Same as Day 2 VS q 8 h	Same as Day 3	Same as Day 4

CLINICAL PATHWAY FOR PNEUMONIA **75**

Skin assessment for color, temp, rashes Anxiety, fear, and fatigue levels; family support and resources Assess response to therapy Monitor for complications • Hypoxemia, dyspnea • Empyema, lung abscess • DVT, PE, pericarditis				
Teaching	Orient to hospital and unit Prepare for diagnostic tests Instruct on use of incentive spirometer, MDI Teach pulmonary hygiene: coughing, positioning, breathing techniques Provide information regarding diagnosis Involve family in care of patient as appropriate Review plan of care/clinical pathway with patient and family	How to recognize and prevent respiratory infection Adaptive breathing techniques: diaphragmatic breathing, staged controlled coughing Positioning for ease of breathing Importance of gradually increasing activity Meds at discharge: action, side effects, time, dosage, route Smoking cessation	Risk factors for and prevention of pneumonia Encourage annual influenza vaccination and pneumococcal vaccine Instruct to call MD for fever, chills, increased cough, dyspnea, chest pain Reinforce Day 2 teaching	Reinforce previous information	Continue as Day 4

Continued

Clinical Pathway for Pneumonia *Continued*

Aspect of Care (Cont'd)	Date ___ Day 1	Date ___ Day 2	Date ___ Day 3	Date ___ Day 4	Date ___ Day 5
Consults	Respiratory therapy	N/A	N/A	N/A	N/A
Lab Tests	ABGs CBC with diff, lytes Blood culture (bacterial pneumonia)	ABGs if pulse ox <90%	Hgb and Hct	N/A	N/A
Other Tests	Chest x-ray: PA and lat Sputum C & S, gram stain	N/A	Chest x-ray if WBC elevated, febrile or abnormal ABGs	N/A	N/A
Meds	Depends on causative organism and sensitivity IV antibiotics: penicillins, cephalosporins, antifungal agents Beta$_2$ agonists q 6 h Bronchodilators via MDI or nebulizer Mucolytics Acetaminophen for temp >101°	Same as Day 1 Change to MDI	Change to PO antibiotics	Same as Day 3	Same as Day 4
Treatments/ Interventions	VS q 4 h Pulse ox q 4 h • O$_2$ per NC if SaO$_2$ <90% Position to facilitate breathing	Same as Day 1 May D/C pulse ox if O$_2$ >94%	Same as Day 2 Incentive spirometer q 4 h W/A	Same as Day 3	Same as Day 4

	Day 1	Day 2	Day 3	Day 4	Day 5
(category label not shown on this page)	• Semi-Fowler's position • Right lung down while on side Incentive spirometry q 4 h Frequent oral care Provide periods of uninterrupted sleep and rest Daily wts Suction if needed Protect from secondary infections (family, visitors with colds)	Same as Day 1	Same as Day 1	Same as Day 3	Same as Day 4
Nutrition	DAT Encourage fluids to 2500 mL/day Assess for decreased appetite	Same as Day 1	Same as Day 2	Same as Day 3	Same as Day 4
Lines/Tubes/Monitors	IV fluids for hydration and medications	Change to saline loc for antibiotics	Same as Day 2	D/C saline loc	N/A
Mobility/Self-Care	OOB to chair as tolerated	OOB and ambulate as tolerated	Same as Day 2	Same as Day 3	Same as Day 4
Discharge Planning	Assist family to modify home environment to reduce fatigue (e.g., avoiding stair climbing)	Continue as Day 1 Ensure teaching plan is followed as discussed above	Continue Day 2	Same as Day 3	Arrange for follow-up visit with MD

Clinical Pathway for Acute Asthma

ICD-9 Code 097   ELOS 3 days

Nursing Diagnosis/ Collaborative Problem	Expected Outcome (The Patient Is Expected to...)	Met/ Not Met	Reason	Date/ Initials
Ineffective breathing pattern	Resume baseline breathing pattern and respiratory rate with a peak flow >70% of baseline			
Ineffective airway clearance	Clear airway without difficulty			
Activity intolerance	Resume activities of daily living with good exercise tolerance			
Ineffective individual and family coping	Identify successful coping strategies and participate in plan of care			

Aspect of Care	Date____ Day 1	Date____ Day 2	Date____ Day 3
Assessment	Systems assessment q shift with focus on respiratory • Adventitious breath sounds and accessory muscle utilization VS q 4 h Sputum for color, tenacity, and amt Skin assessment for color, temp, diaphoresis Anxiety, fear, and fatigue levels; family support and resources	Same as Day 1	Same as Day 2 VS q 8 h

	Assess response to therapy Assess need for mechanical ventilation Monitor for complications • Hypoxemia • Pneumonia • Respiratory acidosis		
Teaching	Orient to hospital and unit Prepare for diagnostic tests Instruct on use of peak expiratory flow meter, nebulizer and MDI Provide information regarding diagnosis and medications Involve family in care of patient as appropriate Review plan of care/clinical pathway with patient and family	Stress reduction techniques, need for adequate rest and sleep How to recognize and prevent respiratory infection, irritants Adaptive breathing techniques (pursed lips, pushing/pulling during exhalation) and energy conserving measures	What to do during acute asthma attack and when to seek emergency care Medication administration and use of MDI Importance of diet and fluids Assess knowledge about factors that trigger asthma and how to pretreat before exposure to trigger Provide information concerning medications that may trigger asthma
Consults	Respiratory therapy Pulmonologist Social worker	N/A	N/A
Lab Tests	CBC with diff, lytes ABGs Theophylline level Total IgE Sputum culture	Theophylline level (while on IV or if dosage changes)	Same as Day 2

Continued

Clinical Pathway for Acute Asthma *Continued*

Aspect of Care (Cont'd)	Date____ Day 1	Date____ Day 2	Date____ Day 3
Other Tests	Chest x-ray ECG (if >40 years of age) Pulmonary function tests	N/A	N/A
Meds	Bronchodilator or beta₂ agonist metaproterenol, albuterol via nebulizer q 4 h *or* IV bronchodilator (aminophylline) via continuous drip Corticosteroids IV q 6 h	Nebulizer q 4 h Consider changing to PO if patient stable Taper dosage and change to PO	Discontinue nebulizer and place on MDI Theo-Dur PO Prednisone PO BID
Treatments/Interventions	O₂ per NC or Ventimask at 2 L to maintain SaO₂ >90% Pulse ox Peak flow before and after nebulizer treatment Bronchodilator via nebulizer or MDI q 4 h Position to facilitate breathing Elevate HOB 45–90° Allergen-free pillow Frequent oral care Provide periods of uninterrupted sleep and rest Daily wts	Same as Day 1	Discontinue O₂ Pulse ox Peak expiratory flow q 8 h Incentive spirometer TID Aerosol inhalation QID Position to facilitate breathing Oral care as needed

Nutrition	DAT (low Na+ if steroid dependent) Encourage fluids to 2000 mL/day (restrict if on steroids)	Same as Day 1	Same as Day 2
Lines/Tubes/Monitors	IV fluids for hydration and medications	Discontinue IV fluids; change to saline loc	Same as Day 2 D/C saline loc
Mobility/Self-Care	Bed rest with BRPs Sit on side of bed or up in bed leaning on overbed table	OOB and ambulate as tolerated	Same as Day 2
Discharge Planning	Assess need for home respiratory equipment	Refer to support group Continue as Day 1 with attention to home needs, modification of environment to reduce allergens	Arrange for follow-up visit with MD

Clinical Pathway for Chronic Airflow Limitation

ICD-9 Code 088   ELOS 5 days

Nursing Diagnosis/ Collaborative Problem	Expected Outcome (The Patient Is Expected to...)	Met/ Not Met	Reason	Date/ Initials
Impaired gas exchange	Maintain blood gases within baseline and use O_2 as appropriate			
Ineffective breathing pattern	Resume baseline breathing pattern and demonstrate correct breathing techniques to decrease work of breathing			
Ineffective airway clearance	Use MDI correctly resulting in a patent airway			
Anxiety	Verbalize feelings about anxiety and use techniques to manage stress			
Activity intolerance and fatigue	Have less fatigue and be able to perform activities of daily living using energy conservation techniques			
Altered nutritional status: Less than body requirements	Maintain current weight and eat balanced diet			

Aspect of Care	Date___ Day 1	Date___ Day 2	Date___ Day 3	Date___ Day 4	Date___ Day 5
Assessment	Systems assessment with focus on respiratory q 4 h • Ability to move secretions • Chest expansion • Adventitious breath sounds • Accessory muscle utilization VS q 4 h Assess for fatigue, anxiety Nutritional and hydration status Sputum for color, odor, consistency, amt Monitor for complications • Hypoxemia • Respiratory acidosis • Cardiac failure and dysrhythmias	Same as Day 1	Same as Day 2 Systems assessment q 8 h VS q 8 h	Same as Day 3	Same as Day 4
Teaching	Orient to hospital and unit Prepare for diagnostic tests Provide information about diagnosis	Continue as Day 1 Teach patient and family postural drainage and percussion/vibration techniques	Teach energy conserving techniques for performing ADLs, breathing techniques, and ways to decrease stress and anxiety	Medication instruction Changes to report to MD • Changes in sputum	Continue as Day 4 Encourage patient to have yearly influenza immunization

Continued

Clinical Pathway for Chronic Airflow Limitation *Continued*

Aspect of Care (Cont'd)	Date____ Day 1	Date____ Day 2	Date____ Day 3	Date____ Day 4	Date____ Day 5
Teaching (Cont'd)	Teach adaptive breathing techniques • Pursed lip, diaphragmatic • Stage-controlled coughing Teach use of MDI Involve family in care of patient as appropriate Review plan of care/clinical pathway with patient and family			• Increased fatigue, SOB, dyspnea • Decreased activity, appetite Importance of adequate diet and fluid intake Provide information regarding exposure to environmental irritants	
Consults	Dietician Pulmonologist Respiratory therapist Social worker	Rehab services: PT/OT	N/A	N/A	N/A
Lab Tests	ABGs Sputum for C & S, gram stain CBC with diff, lytes, BUN, Cr Serum protein, albumin Theophylline level (if taking at home)	Check sputum results and modify treatment if indicated	N/A	Lytes, BUN, Cr Theophylline level	N/A

	Day 1	Day 2	Day 3	Day 4	Day 5
Other Tests	Chest x-ray Pulmonary function tests • Vital capacity • Residual volume • Total lung capacity • Flow volume curves ECG	N/A	N/A	N/A	N/A
Meds	Antibiotics according to sensitivity IV q 6 h Continuous IV aminophylline IV corticosteroid q 6 h MDI q 4 h Bronchodilator via nebulizer q 4–6 h	Continue as Day 1 Taper steroids	D/C IV meds and change to PO MDI PRN	Same as Day 3	Same as Day 4
Treatments/ Interventions	I & O O_2 per NC 1–2 L/min Pulse ox Position to facilitate breathing • Semi-Fowler's Suction as needed Daily wts	Same as Day 1 Respiratory muscle training, breathing exercises, and exercise conditioning	Same as Day 2	Same as Day 3	Same as Day 4
Nutrition	Diet as tolerated Encourage fluids to 2 L/day if tolerated	Same as Day 1	Same as Day 2	Same as Day 3	Same as Day 4

Continued

Clinical Pathway for Chronic Airflow Limitation *Continued*

Aspect of Care (Cont'd)	Date____ Day 1	Date____ Day 2	Date____ Day 3	Date____ Day 4	Date____ Day 5
Lines/Tubes/ Monitors	Saline loc for IV meds	Same as Day 1	Discontinue saline loc	N/A	N/A
Mobility/Self-Care	Bed rest with BRPs or sitting on edge of bed with arms folded on pillows on bedside table	OOB and ambulate as tolerated	Same as Day 2	Same as Day 3	Same as Day 4
Discharge Planning	Assess need for social services, financial status, health insurance and coverage, home environment, need for placement and family support Assess need for home respiratory equipment	Arrange for home O$_2$ and respiratory therapy if needed	Continue as Day 2	Refer to smokers cessation program if appropriate Ensure that all equipment is at home and functioning Refer to pulmonary rehab	Arrange for follow-up visit with MD

Notes

Unit

II

Problems of Circulation/ Cardiovascular Health Problems

▼ ▼ ▼

Clinical Pathway for Uncomplicated Myocardial Infarction

ICD-9 Code 410.91   ELOS 4 days

Nursing Diagnosis/ Collaborative Problem	Expected Outcome (The Patient Is Expected to...)	Met/ Not Met	Reason	Date/ Initials
Pain	State that chest pain is relieved			
Altered tissue perfusion (cardiopulmonary)	Have resolution of ST and T wave changes and pulse ox reading of >90%; have clear breath sounds			
Activity intolerance	Ambulate in hall without experiencing extreme fatigue or chest pain			
Ineffective individual and family coping	Verbalize feelings about having an MI and future fears; identify effective coping strategies			
Potential for heart failure	Not experience ventricular dysfunction, dysrhythmia, or crackles			

Aspect of Care	Date ___ Day 1 (CCU)	Date ___ Day 2 (CCU)	Date ___ Day 3 (Telemetry)	Date ___ Day 4 (Telemetry)
Assessment	Chest pain assessment with VS q 1–2 h Cardiac monitoring Assess for related S/S, such as dyspnea, diaphoresis, nausea	Chest pain assessment with VS q 4 h if stable Cardiac monitoring Assess for S/S of heart failure	Same as Day 1 Assessment for transfer to telemetry or progressive cardiac unit	VS q 8 h; chest pain assessment Cardiac monitoring

	Assess for coping ability/anxiety level; Risk factor assessment, such as smoking history, diet, activity, family history, lipid profile; Systems assessment q 8 h; Mental status assessment QD; Code status/advance directives; If received thrombolytics, assess for S/S of bleeding	Teaching/learning ability assessment; assess for barriers to learning		
Teaching	Orient to hospital and unit; Explain procedures and treatments carefully; Teach importance of reporting chest pain or unusual sensations; Review plan of care/clinical pathway with patient and family	Begin cardiac teaching; review MI diagnosis; teach need for activity restriction/energy conservation	Continue with cardiac teaching • Meds, diet, weight monitoring; Orient to telemetry unit	Review discharge instructions regarding: • Chest pain occurrence • Meds • Diet • Physical activity progression • Sexual activity • Reduction of risk factors (smoking cessation, exercise, diet)
Consults	Cardiologist, if indicated; Cardiac rehab; Social worker for discharge planning	Dietician	PT, if needed for increasing mobility	N/A
Lab Tests	CBC, lytes, Mg^{+2}, BUN, Cr, glucose (SMA-6 or 6/60); Cardiac enzymes q 8–12 h	SMA-6 or 6/60; Repeat enzymes if elevated	Same as Day 2	N/A

Continued

Clinical Pathway for Uncomplicated Myocardial Infarction *Continued*

Aspect of Care (Cont'd)	Date ___ Day 1 (CCU)	Date ___ Day 2 (CCU)	Date ___ Day 3 (Telemetry)	Date ___ Day 4 (Telemetry)
Lab Tests (Cont'd)	INR(PT)/APTT ABGs, pulse ox, as indicated	INR(PT/APTT), if on anticoagulant therapy	N/A	N/A
Other Tests	ECG Chest x-ray	Echocardiogram/MUGA scan (may be done on Day 1)	Cardiac cath, if needed	ECG Stress test (per MD preference)
Meds	Thrombolytic therapy, if meets criteria Analgesic (usually morphine) Stool softener Lidocaine drip, as indicated Nitrates and/or inotropes, as indicated (IV, PO, or topical) Anticoagulant (heparin, Coumadin or ASA) Beta blocker/calcium channel blocker ACE inhibitor	Same as Day 1, except for thrombolytic therapy	Switch to PO analgesics as needed Stool softener PO or topical nitrates Anticoagulant Beta blocker/calcium channel block ACE inhibitor	Anticoagulant Beta blocker/calcium channel blocker Nitrate Stool softener ACE inhibitor
Treatments/ Interventions	O₂ 2–4 L via NC (maintain O₂ saturation >90%) I & O Daily wt, as indicated Emotional support: encourage ventilation of feelings about MI	Same as Day 1	Transfer to telemetry or progressive cardiac unit per assessment Same as Day 1	O₂ 2 L via NC Continue with emotional support D/C daily wt unless patient has CHF

Nutrition	Progressive cardiac diet (2–4 GM Na+, ↓ fat if ↑ serum lipids)	Same as Day 1	Same as Day 2	Cardiac diet
Lines/Tubes/Monitors	Continuous IV fluids (monitor for fluid overload) Cardiac monitor (CCU)	Same as Day 1	Convert IV to saline loc Same as Day 1 (telemetry)	D/C saline loc Telemetry
Mobility/Self-Care	Bed rest with BSC Assist with ADLs, as needed	Cardiac rehab protocol; up in chair 30 min x 3/day Assist with ADLs as needed	BRP and ambulate in room if ambulatory	Ambulate in hall, if able, with supervision per cardiac rehab protocol
Discharge Planning	Assess home needs and family support/resources	Collaborate with social worker to determine disposition: home, NH, other	Contact/refer to home health services, if needed, for discharge to home (may need homemaker, nursing, PT to increase activity tolerance)	Arrange for follow-up appointment with MD per order Arrange for stress test as outpatient, as specified per MD

Clinical Pathway for Congestive Heart Failure

ICD-9 Code 428.0   ELOS 5 days

Nursing Diagnosis/Collaborative Problem	Expected Outcome (The Patient Is Expected to...)	Met/Not Met	Reason	Date/Initials
Decreased cardiac output/fluid volume overload	Have a heart rate within baseline, no significant dependent edema, clear lungs, BP within baseline, and no neck vein distention			
Impaired gas exchange	Have ABGs WNL and respiratory rate within normal rate, rhythm, and depth with equal expansion and breath sounds			
Fatigue/activity intolerance	Perform ADLs without experiencing shortness of breath			
Potential for life-threatening dysrhythmias	Be free of life-threatening dysrhythmias; have normal sinus rhythm			

Aspect of Care	Date____ Day 1	Date____ Day 2	Date____ Day 3	Date____ Day 4	Date____ Day 5
Assessment	Systems assessment; Code status/advance directives; Chest pain assessment with VS	VS q 4 h; Chest pain assessment with VS; Breath sounds q 8 h	VS q 4–8 h, as indicated; Chest pain and mental status; Breath sounds q 8 h	VS q 8 h; Continue to monitor breath sounds q 8 h; Mental status assessment	Same as Day 4

Assessment (cont.)	VS q 1–4 h, as indicated Mental status assessment QD Breath sounds q 8 h	Teaching/learning ability assessment; assess barriers to learning		Chest pain assessment	
Teaching	Orient to hospital and unit Review plan of care/clinical pathway with patient and family Explain procedures and treatments carefully Teach importance of reporting chest pain or unusual sensations	Review CHF diagnosis Teach need for activity restriction/energy conservation	Begin teaching about cardiac meds, special diet, and wt monitoring	Continue with teaching/provide discharge instructions regarding: • Activity restrictions • Dietary/fluid restrictions • Meds (administration, side effects) • When to notify MD of significant changes such as swelling of hands and feet or sudden weight gain Provide written materials from the American Heart Association	Review discharge instructions as listed on Day 4
Consults	Cardiologist, if needed Dietician Social worker	Cardiac rehab OT for ADLs, if needed	N/A	N/A	N/A

Continued

Clinical Pathway for Congestive Heart Failure Continued

Aspect of Care (Cont'd)	Date ___ Day 1	Date ___ Day 2	Date ___ Day 3	Date ___ Day 4	Date ___ Day 5
Lab Tests	CBC, lytes, Mg^{+2} BUN, Cr, glucose (SMA-6 or 6/60) Cardiac enzymes q 8–12 h Digitalis level, if indicated ABGs, pulse ox, as ordered INR(PT)/APTT	Same as Day 1 Cardiac enzymes, if elevated INR(PT)/APTT QD if on anticoagulants	Same as Day 2	Repeat tests, as indicated Digtalis level	N/A
Other Tests	ECG Chest x-ray	ECG MUGA scan or echocardiogram	ECG	ECG, if indicated	N/A
Meds	Review med regimen before admission Digoxin Lasix (or other loop diuretic) IV push or PO as needed K$^+$ supplement, if low K$^+$ ACE inhibitor Anticoagulant, if clotting disorder or prophylactically Nitrates and/or inotropes (IV, PO, or topical)	Same as Day 1	Same as Day 2	Continue with meds PO	Same as Day 4

	Day 1	Day 2	Day 3	Day 4	Day 5
Treatments/ Interventions	Telemetry, if severe dysrhythmias; O_2 via NC, as needed; Daily wts (before breakfast); Strict I & O	Same as Day 1	Same as Day 2; Assess for transfer from telemetry	O_2 via NC, as needed; Daily wts (before breakfast); Strict I & O	Same as Day 4
Nutrition	Fluid restriction; Low sodium diet (NAS → 2 GM Na^+) per MD/dietician	Same as Day 1	Same as Day 2	Fluid restriction, if needed; Low sodium diet	Same as Day 4
Lines/Tubes/ Monitors	Saline loc or IV fluids at KVO rate	Saline loc	Same as Day 2	Saline loc	D/C saline loc
Mobility/Self-Care	Bed rest; Total care	Bed rest or BRPs/BSC with assistance, if no dyspnea; May be up in chair for 10–15 min with assistance per MD; Assist with ADLs as needed	May ambulate in room with assistance, if ambulatory; Provide frequent rest periods; Assist with ADLs as needed	Ambulate in room; may need assistance (walker or helper); Provide frequent rest periods	Same as Day 4
Discharge Planning	Assess home needs and family support/resources (focus on physical environment, e.g., stairs, location of bathroom)	Collaborate with social worker to determine disposition: home or NH	Same as Day 2	Assess need for referral to home health services (if discharged to home), including homemaker, nursing, OT/PT to increase activity tolerance	Arrange for follow-up appointment with MD per order

Clinical Pathway for Peripheral Arterial Revascularization (Bypass Graft)

ICD-9 Code 440.21/39.29   ELOS 4 days

Nursing Diagnosis/ Collaborative Problem	Expected Outcome (The Patient Is Expected to...)	Met/ Not Met	Reason	Date/ Initials
Potential for acute altered tissue perfusion (graft occlusion)	Have warm lower extremities with palpable pulses			
Potential for hemorrhage or wound infection	Have Hgb, Hct, and WBC WNL; have clean and dry surgical incisions			
Pain	State that pain in lower extremity is reduced or alleviated by surgery and appropriate pain management techniques			

Aspect of Care	Date____ Pre-Admission/Pre-op	Date____ Day 1 (DOS)	Date____ Day 2 (POD #1)	Date____ Day 3 (POD #2)	Date____ Day 4 (POD #3)
Assessment	Systems assessment Psychosocial assessment Pre-op checklist	*PACU:* VS q 15 min x 4, q 30 min x 4 with LE circulation checks (use Doppler, if needed, to check pedal pulses), mark pedal pulse point Systems assessment Pain assessment, especially location of pain	VS q 4 h with LE circulation checks Systems assessment, especially breath sounds and skin Pain assessments Monitor dressings	VS q 4 h with circulation checks Systems assessment Monitor incisions for drainage; keep covered if oozing Assess for BM Check heels for breakdown	VS q 8 h with circulation checks Systems assessment Monitor incisions Check heels

	Monitor dressings for drainage *Post-op:* VS q 1 h x 4, then q 4 h if stable Circulation checks of LE with VS (notify MD of change) Systems assessment Pain assessment Monitor surgical dressings				
Teaching	Review clinical pathway/plan of care with patient and family Reinforce surgical procedure Review post-op expectations, such as DB & C, pain managment, incision care, anticoagulant therapy Orient to hospital and unit	Reinforce DB & C/ incentive spirometer Remind patient to report extreme leg pain or numbness	Teach patient to keep surgical leg straight and elevated while OOB Teach patient to avoid crossing legs or ankles	Teach discharge instructions regarding • Wound care • Pain management • Bleeding precautions • Follow-up lab work • Activity restrictions	Review discharge teaching per Day 3
Consults	Cardiologist, if history of cardiac disease	N/A	PT for walker instruction Social worker for placement, if needed	N/A	N/A
Lab Tests	Routine admission tests, including CBC with diff, SMA-6, Cr, INR(PT)/APTT	INR(PT)/APTT	Hgb and Hct INR(PT)/APTT	INR(PT)/APTT	INR(PT)/APTT

Continued

Clinical Pathway for Peripheral Arterial Revascularization (Bypass Graft) *Continued*

Aspect of Care (Cont'd)	Date_____ Pre-Admission/Pre-op	Date_____ Day 1 (DOS)	Date_____ Day 2 (POD #1)	Date_____ Day 3 (POD #2)	Date_____ Day 4 (POD #3)
Other Tests	Vascular studies ECG, chest x-ray	N/A	N/A	N/A	N/A
Meds	IV antibiotic prior to OR and/or during OR Pre-anesthesia meds D/C aspirin, NSAIDs, and other drugs that increase bleeding times	IV antibiotics for prophylaxis every 6–8 h x 24 h Heparin continuous infusion Stool softener at bedtime PCA or IM morphine or meperidine (Demerol)	D/C PCA Continue with heparin infusion Begin Coumadin therapy per lab results IM or PO opioid analgesia as needed q 3–4 h for pain Stool softener at bedtime	Continue with Coumadin and PO analgesic, such as Tylox q 3–4 h PRN Stool softener at bedtime Laxative of choice, if needed	Same as Day 3
Treatments/ Interventions	Betadine scrub to surgical leg	Antiembolism stocking to nonsurgical leg Pressure dressing with ace wrap to surgical leg DB & C q 2 h W/A with incentive spirometer Turning allowance ordered by MD Keep heels off bed Bed cradle for comfort I & O while on IVs	Same as Day 1	Clean incisions with NS at least BID Maintain antiembolism stockings/ace wrap	Same as Day 3
Nutrition	NPO after 12 midnight the day before surgery	Ice chips/clear liquids (small amount) if no nausea and early AM surgery	Clear liquids → progress DAT	DAT	Same as Day 3

Lines/Tubes/Monitors	IV with 18g cath Foley cath during OR only	Continuous IV fluids	D/C IV fluids, except heparin	D/C IV; convert to saline loc	D/C saline loc
Mobility/Self-Care	Ad lib	Bed rest (turn per MD order) Do not raise HOB >15° (avoid hip flexion)	Up with assistance to chair BID Avoid extreme hip flexion and do not bend surgical knee (keep patient's leg straight) Elevate surgical leg while OOB	Up with walker to bathroom in room Keep leg as straight as possible Elevate surgical leg when sitting Avoid sitting for prolonged periods	Up with walker into hall Keep leg straight and elevate Avoid prolonged sitting
Discharge Planning	N/A	N/A	Evaluate home support systems and feasibility of direct discharge to home If NH placement needed, begin arrangements	Make arrangements for home health services if discharged to home and has minimal support system	Make follow-up appointment with MD, as specified, for home discharge

Unit
III

Problems of Motor and Sensory Function/Neurologic Health Problems

▼ ▼ ▼

Clinical Pathway for Lumbar Laminectomy with Fusion

ICD-9 Code 214   ELOS 4 days

Nursing Diagnosis/Collaborative Problem	Expected Outcome (The Patient Is Expected to...)	Met/Not Met	Reason	Date/Initials
Potential for neurologic deficit	Have a neuro status WNL, positive pedal pulses, and normal sensory status			
Pain	State that pain is relieved and muscle spasms reduced after appropriate interventions			
Impaired physical mobility	Ambulate in hall independently and follow appropriate body mechanics and post-op restrictions (no lifting or twisting)			

Aspect of Care	Date ___ Pre-admission/Pre-	Date ___ Day 1 (DOS)	Date ___ Day 2 (POD #1)	Date ___ Day 3 (POD #2)	Date ___ Day 4 (POD #3)
Assessment	Systems assessment with attention to neuro status: movement, sensation Pre-op check list NV check Document use of nonsteroid anti-inflammatory meds Psychosocial assessment	*PACU:* VS and NV checks q 15 min x 4 then q 30 min x 2 Systems and pain assessment Check incision and Hemovac/JP for drainage and patency	VS and NV checks q 4 h Systems assessment q 8 h Pain assessment Check dressings for drainage Monitor for complications • CSF leak • Paralytic ileus	Same as Day 2 Check incisions for S/S of infection Assess ability to perform ADLs	VS and NV checks q 8 h Systems assessment q 8 h Pain assessment

Skin assessment and temp	*Post-op:* VS and NV checks q 1 h x 4 then q 4 h Systems assessment q 8 h Pain assessment Check lumbar and iliac dressing for drainage Check Hemovac/JP for drainage Monitor for complications • CSF leak • Paralytic ileus • Muscle spasms • Urinary retention • Headache	• Infection • Urinary retention • Muscle spasms • Headache		
Teaching	Orient to hospital and post-op routine • Logrolling techniques • Body mechanics and alignment • Techniques to get in and out of bed • Breathing exercises Explain how bone graft will be obtained Pain control techniques	Involve family in care of patient as appropriate Review plan of care/clinical pathway with patient and family	Instruct patient not to twist, flex, hyper-extend, pull on side rails Instruct on body mechanics, muscle strengthening exercises	Same as Day 2 S/S of infection Care of incision sites Activity restrictions (no heavy lifting, sitting for prolonged periods of time)	Same as Day 3
Consults	Medical clearance	Social worker	PT/OT	N/A	N/A

Continued

Clinical Pathway for Lumbar Laminectomy with Fusion *Continued*

Aspect of Care (Cont'd)	Date ___ Pre-admission/Pre-op	Date ___ Day 1 (DOS)	Date ___ Day 2 (POD #1)	Date ___ Day 3 (POD #2)	Date ___ Day 4 (POD #3)
Lab Tests	CT/MRI Lumbar spine films CBC with diff, lytes Type and screen INR(PT)/APTT	N/A	Hgb & Hct	N/A	CBC with diff, lytes
Other Tests	Chest x-ray ECG (if >40 years old)	N/A	N/A	N/A	N/A
Meds	Antibiotic (e.g., Ancef, vancomycin) IV before surgery	*PACU:* Analgesia IM, epidural cath or PCA pump morphine if patient awake and stable *Post-op:* Continue analgesia as above Antibiotic IV q 6 h x 48 h	Continue epidural cath or PCA pump or change to oral analgesia (Tylenol #3, codeine) Stool softener (Colace) TID	D/C epidural cath or PCA pump Oral analgesia Stool softener	Change to Tylenol PO PRN
Treatments/ Interventions	Thigh-high antiembolism stockings Emotional support	Thigh-high antiembolism stockings and SCDs TCDB q 2 h Incentive spirometer q 2 h W/A I & O	Same as Day 1	Same as Day 2	Same as Day 3

Nutrition	NPO after 12 midnight	*Post-op:* NPO until 4 h after surgery then ice chips/clear liquids and advance as tolerated	DAT	DAT	Same as Day 3
Lines/Tubes/Monitors	N/A	Continuous IV fluids. Check drainage from hemovac/JP drain • Measure and record output. Foley to straight drainage	IV fluids to KVO or to saline loc. Check drainage from hemovac/JP • Measure and record output	Hemovac/JP removed. Saline loc removed. D/C Foley	N/A
Mobility/Self-Care	Bed rest with BRPs	Bed rest. Logroll q 2 hr	OOB to chair as tolerated with lumbar brace. Begin leg exercises	OOB with lumbar brace. Ambulate as tolerated	OOB and ambulate with brace as tolerated
Discharge Planning	Identify need for home modifications. Discuss work restrictions and time off and financial implications	Same as pre-admission	Instruct family to obtain firm mattress or place bed board under mattress. Review activity restrictions. Obtain any assistive/adaptive devices, if needed	Same as Day 2	Review discharge instructions. Arrange for follow-up appointment with MD

Clinical Pathway for Cervical Laminectomy with Fusion

ICD-9 Code 722.0/80.51, 81.02   ELOS 3 days

Nursing Diagnosis/ Collaborative Problem	Expected Outcome (The Patient Is Expected to...)	Met/ Not Met	Reason	Date/ Initials
Potential for neurologic deficit	Have minimal or no residual motor or sensory impairment			
Pain	State that pain is relieved after appropriate interventions			
Impaired physical mobility	Ambulate in hall independently and follow appropriate body mechanics and post-op restrictions (lifting, twisting)			

Aspect of Care	Date____ Pre-admission/Pre-op	Date____ Day 1 (DOS)	Date____ Day 2 (POD #1)	Date____ Day 3 (POD #2)
Assessment	Systems assessment with attention to neuro status • Arm movement, sensation, ROM, reflexes Pre-op check list Psychosocial assessment Skin assessment for color, temp	*PACU:* VS and NV checks q 15 min x 4 then q 30 min x 2 Systems and pain assessment *Post-op:* VS and NV checks q 1 h x 4 then q 4 h Systems and pain assessment Check cervical and iliac dressing for drainage	VS and NV checks q 4 h Systems assessment q shift Pain assessment Check dressings for drainage Check incisions for S/S of infection	Same as Day 2 Assess ability to perform ADLs

Teaching	Orient to hospital and post-op routine • Body mechanics and alignment • Techniques to get in and out of bed • Breathing exercises Explain pain management Explain how bone graft will be obtained	Monitor for complications • CSF leak • Neuro status change • Respiratory changes Involve family in care of patient as appropriate Review plan of care/clinical pathway with patient and family	Instruct patient not to twist, flex, hyperextend, pull on side rails Instruct on body mechanics, muscle strengthening exercises Teach importance of wearing cervical collar	Same as Day 2 S/S of infection Care of incision sites Activity restrictions (no heavy lifting, sitting for prolonged periods of time)
Consults	Social worker	N/A	N/A	N/A
Lab Tests	CBC with diff, lytes Type and screen U/A INR(PT)/APPT	N/A	Hgb & Hct, lytes	N/A
Other Tests	Chest x-ray ECG (if >40 years old or history of cardiac disease)	N/A	N/A	C-spine: PA and lateral
Meds	Antibiotic (cefazolin, cefamandole) IV before surgery	*PACU:* Analgesia IM or PCA pump morphine if patient awake and stable *Post-op:* Same as PACU Antibiotics	Change to oral analgesia Assess need for stool softener	Same as Day 2

Continued

Clinical Pathway for Cervical Laminectomy with Fusion *Continued*

Aspect of Care (Cont'd)	Date _____ Pre-admission/Pre-op	Date _____ Day 1 (DOS)	Date _____ Day 2 (POD #1)	Date _____ Day 3 (POD #2)
Treatments/ Interventions	Thigh-high antiembolism stockings Emotional support	Thigh-high antiembolism stockings or SCDs TCDB q 2 h Incentive spirometer q 4 h I & O	Same as Day 1	Thigh-high antiembolism stockings D/C incentive spirometer D/C I & O
Nutrition	NPO after 12 midnight	NPO until 6 h after surgery then ice chips/clear liquids	Clear liquids, advance as tolerated	DAT
Lines/Tubes/Monitors	N/A	Continuous IV fluids	D/C IV fluids; change to saline loc if tolerating PO fluids D/C PCA pump	D/C saline loc
Mobility/Self-Care	BRPs	Bed rest with BSC Logroll q 2 h	OOB as tolerated to chair with cervical collar	OOB and ambulate as tolerated with cervical collar
Discharge Planning	Identify need for home modification or assistive/ adaptive devices	Continue as pre-admission	Continue as Day 1 Review activity restrictions	Continue as Day 2 Arrange for follow-up visit with MD

Notes

Clinical Pathway for Cerebral Vascular Accident (CVA)

ICD-9 Code 014   ELOS 4 days

Nursing Diagnosis/ Collaborative Problem	Expected Outcome (The Patient Is Expected to...)	Met/ Not Met	Reason	Date/ Initials
Altered cerebral tissue perfusion	Maintain baseline vital and neuro signs			
Sensory perceptual alteration	Have minimal complications and remain free of injury			
	Be oriented to environment			
Impaired physical mobility	Ambulate with or without assistive/adaptive devices			
Self-care deficit	Perform own self-care with or without assistive/adaptive devices			
	Family member has received instruction on how to assist the patient			
Impaired verbal communication	Utilize communication strategies via speaking, communication board, or voice synthesizer			
Impaired swallowing	Eat meals without aspiration			
	Have an adequate nutritional status			

Aspect of Care	Date ___ Day 1	Date ___ Day 2	Date ___ Day 3	Date ___ Day 4
Assessment	Systems assessment with attention to neuro and cardiovascular system • Change in LOC • Visual field deficit • Cognitive and language deficit • Cranial nerve deficit • Heart sounds and rhythm Evaluate need for Foley cath VS and NS q 4 h Monitor for complications • Aspiration • Paralytic ileus • DVT, PE, SIADH, DI • Atrial fibrillation, dysrhythmias • Increased ICP, hydro-cephalus Monitor for bleeding if on anticoagulant	Same as Day 1 Systems assessment q 8 h Assess pulmonary status before and after meals for aspiration pneumonia Assess for risk of falling	Same as Day 2 Assess for depression and emotional lability	Same as Day 3 VS q 8 h
Teaching	Orient to unit and hospital Prepare for diagnostic tests Provide information about diagnosis Involve family in care of patient as appropriate Review care plan/critical pathway with patient and family	Prepare for diagnostic tests Continue education regarding diagnosis Begin ADL training • Communication • Visual field deficits • Muscle strengthening • Swallowing	Same as Day 2 Begin bowel and bladder program, if incontinent Teach lifestyle modification • Diet • Exercise • Quit smoking	Same as Day 3 Instruct regarding meds to be administered at home • Route, time, action, side effects

Continued

Clinical Pathway for Cerebral Vascular Accident (CVA) *Continued*

Aspect of Care (Cont'd)	Date___ Day 1	Date___ Day 2	Date___ Day 3	Date___ Day 4
Teaching (Cont'd)		Continue family involvement *Right hemisphere stroke:* Teach to scan to left side. Have visitors sit on patient's left side, provide tactile stimulation to left side. Eliminate distraction of TV/radio *Left hemisphere stroke:* Communication skills		
Consults	Dietician Neurologist Social worker	Rehab services: PT/OT/SLP Swallowing evaluation	N/A	N/A
Lab Tests	CBC with diff U/A Coag studies Serum electrolytes ESR	APTT, if on heparin Serum albumin, total protein	APTT, if on heparin INR(PT), if on oral anticoagulants	INR(PT)
Other Tests	CT/MRI Chest x-ray ECG Cerebral angiogram if hemorrhagic stroke	Ultrasonic or Doppler study *Embolic stroke:* • Echocardiogram • Holter monitor EEG	N/A	N/A

Meds	*If cause other than hemorrhagic stroke:* • Heparin continuous infusion • ASA one tab or dipyridamole Anticonvulsant Calcium channel blocker, if stroke due to subarachnoid hemorrhage Antihypertensive Diuretic Opioid or nonopioid analgesic	Same as Day 1	Change heparin to oral anticoagulant	Same as Day 3
Treatments/ Interventions	Strict I & O Elevate HOB 30 to 45° Thigh-high antiembolism stockings Seizure precautions Daily wts Place call light in easy reach Suction as needed Mouth care q shift Develop communication system Prevent from injury Speak slowly, using short, simple sentences	Same as Day 1	Same as Day 2	I & O Thigh-high antiembolism stockings Elevate HOB 15–30° Continue with communication system Prevent from injury and falls

Continued

Clinical Pathway for Cerebral Vascular Accident (CVA) Continued

Aspect of Care (Cont'd)	Date ____ Day 1	Date ____ Day 2	Date ____ Day 3	Date ____ Day 4
Nutrition	NPO	DAT • Check for swallowing deficit • Semisolid or pureed Assist with meals • HOB elevated 90° • Tilt head slightly forward • Use spoon	Same as Day 2	Same as Day 3
Lines/Tubes/Monitors	Continuous IV fluids Monitor for dehydration or overhydration	Same as Day 1	Convert IV to saline loc	D/C saline loc
Mobility/Self-Care	Bed rest TCDB q 2 h Active or passive ROM to all extremities q 4 h Maintain body alignment and support extremities with pillows, minimize stress on joints Skin assessment and care Use footboard, boots to prevent foot drop	*Same as Day 1 except:* OOB to chair TID • Monitor for hypotension Arm sling to affected arm Muscle strengthening program Use assistive/adaptive devices for ambulation/transfers	*Same as Day 2 except:* Begin ambulation as tolerated with assistive devices as needed	Same as Day 3

Discharge Planning		
Social worker to assess need for social services, financial status, health insurance and coverage, home environment, need for placement, and family support	Identify placement for discharge • Rehab facility • ECF • Home	Begin discharge instruction and notes for ECF or rehab facility *or* Ensure that home has been equipped with assistive/adaptive devices and that family and patient know how to use them	Continue as Day 3 Arrange for follow-up visit with MD

Unit

IV

Problems of Mobility/ Musculoskeletal Health Problems

▼ ▼ ▼

Clinical Pathway for Hip Open Reduction, Internal Fixation (ORIF)

ICD-9 Code 820.8/81.51   ELOS 7 days

Nursing Diagnosis/ Collaborative Problem	Expected Outcome (The Patient Is Expected to...)	Met/ Not Met	Reason	Date/ Initials
Pain	State that pain is relieved following appropriate interventions (if cognitively intact); not be restless or agitated			
Potential for neurovascular compromise of affected extremity	Have warm LE with pulses present			
Acute confusion	Participate in self-care activities (if able to do ADLs independently before fracture)			
Impaired physical mobility	Ambulate with walker in room (if ambulatory before fracture); not experience complications of immobility			
Potential for postoperative complications (hip dislocation, hemorrhage, infection, thromboembolitic complications)	Not experience hip dislocation; have Hgb and Hct WNL, stable VS, WBC WNL, and no S/S of DVT, PE, or other thromboembolitic complications			

Aspect of Care	Date _____ Day 1 (Day of Admission)	Date _____ Day 2 (DOS)	Date _____ Day 3 (POD #1)	Date _____ Day 4 (POD #2)	Date _____ Day 5 (POD #3)	Date _____ Day 6–7 (POD #4–5)
Assessment	VS and NV check q 4 h and PRN	Complete pre-op checklist	VS and NV checks q 4 h	VS and NV checks q 8 h	Same as Day 4 (POD #2)	Same as Day 5 (POD #3)
	Systems assessment	*PACU:*	Systems assessment with focus on breath and bowel sounds, skin assessment, mentation, pain	Monitor incision for S/S of infection		
	Pain assessment	VS q 15 min x 4, q 30 min x 4		Systems assessment		
	Mental status evaluation; compare with pre-admission baseline if able	NV checks with VS	Keep hip abducted	Pain assessment		
	Skin assessment	Check hip dressing and drain	Check hip dressing and drain q 8 h	Monitor mental status		
	Assess anxiety level	Check hip alignment (abduction)	Check voiding	Assess for BM		
		Systems assessment				
		Pain and mental status assessment				
		Post-op:				
		VS q 1 h x 4, then q 4 h if stable; NV checks with VS				
		Check hip dressing and measure wound drainage q 8 h				
		Check voiding, if no Foley				
		Assess skin, especially heels				

Continued

Clinical Pathway for Hip Open Reduction, Internal Fixation (ORIF) Continued

Aspect of Care (Cont'd)	Date____ Day 1 (Day of Admission)	Date____ Day 2 (DOS)	Date____ Day 3 (POD #1)	Date____ Day 4 (POD #2)	Date____ Day 5 (POD #3)	Date____ Day 6–7 (POD #4–5)
Teaching	Orient to hospital and unit Provide/reinforce pre-op teaching to patient/family regarding • Incision • Procedure • Pain management • Hip precautions • Post-op expectations	Reinforce teaching from Day 1 Teach purpose of meds Teach/demonstrate DB & C technique, incentive spirometer	Teach/demonstrate procedure for ankle pumps, quad and gluteal sets Teach additional pain relief measures, such as imagery, if appropriate (patient is not cognitively impaired)	Reinforce teaching from previous days	Begin discharge teaching regarding • Wound care • Pain management • Physical activity • Exercises • Complications • Meds • Hip precautions • Bleeding precautions/testing • Rehab program	Continue with discharge teaching
Consults	Social worker Respiratory therapy, if available	N/A	PT for evaluation and rehab potential Dietician, if underweight or low albumin/transferrin	N/A	N/A	N/A
Lab Tests	CBC with diff, SMA-6 (6/60), type and crossmatch, INR(PT)/APTT, albumin/transferrin	Hct in AM	Hct in AM Daily INR(PT)/APTT	Daily INR(PT)/APTT	Same as Day 4 (POD #2)	Same as Day 5 (POD #3)
Other Tests	Chest x-ray ECG Hip x-ray	Post-op x-ray of affected hip	N/A	N/A	N/A	N/A

Meds	PO or IM meperidine or morphine (give with low-dose Vistaril to ↓ anxiety)	IM or PCA meperidine or morphine (if ↑ confusion, D/C PCA)	Same as Day 2 (DOS)	IM or PO opioids (meperidine or morphine for IM; Percocet [Tylox] PO PRN q 3–4 h	Switch to PO opioids	Same as Day 5 (POD #3)
	Continue with baseline meds, as indicated	Antiemetic PRN	Calcium/vitamin D supplements, if severe osteoporosis	Continue with ordered anticoagulant based on daily INR(PT)/APTT	Anticoagulant	
	Prophylactic antibiotic (cephalosporin)	Heparin SQ, Lovenox, or Coumadin for anticoagulation		Stool softener	Stool softener	
		Tylenol q 3–4 h PRN for temp >100°F or pain		Tylenol PRN	Tylenol	
		Stool softener at bedtime		Calcium/vitamin D supplements for severe osteoporosis	Laxative of choice PRN	
		Antibiotic IV PB (cephalosporin) q 6–8 h x 3–4 doses			Calcium/vitamin D supplement for severe osteoporosis	
Treatments/ Interventions	Buck's traction	I & O	Same as Day 2 (DOS)	Antiembolism stockings	Antiembolism stockings	Same as Day 5 (POD #3)
	Antiembolism stockings (thigh-high, if tolerated)	Antiembolism stockings	D/C I & O if IV D/C'd and voiding is adequate	SCDs while in bed	SCDs while in bed	
	SCDs	SCDs		DB & C q 2 h W/A; incentive spirometer	DB & C; incentive spirometer	
	I & O	Pillow or other abduction device in place		Abduction device/pillow at night	Abduction device/pillow at night	
	Betadine scrub to affected hip area	TCDB q 2 h W/A (turn to unaffected side but keep legs abducted)		MD to change or remove hip dressing/drain	Clean incision BID with NS, cover with sterile gauze if draining	
	ROM to unaffected LE and UE	Incentive spirometer q 2 h W/A; O2 PRN		Clean incision BID with NS; cover with sterile gauze if draining		
	O2 via NC if O2 saturation <90%	Nebulizer treatment if pulmonary history				

Continued

Clinical Pathway for Hip Open Reduction, Internal Fixation (ORIF) *Continued*

Aspect of Care (Cont'd)	Date _____ Day 1 (Day of Admission)	Date _____ Day 2 (DOS)	Date _____ Day 3 (POD #1)	Date _____ Day 4 (POD #2)	Date _____ Day 5 (POD #3)	Date _____ Day 6–7 (POD #4–5)
Nutrition	DAT (unless on restrictions PTA) NPO after 12 midnight	NPO pre-op Clear → full liquids post-op	DAT (unless on restrictions PTA) May need supplement such as Ensure, per dietician consult	Same as Day 3 (POD #1)	Same as Day 4 (POD #2)	Same as Day 5 (POD #3)
Lines/Tubes/Monitors	IV with 18g cath Foley cath to straight drainage	Same as Day 1 (Foley may be removed after OR) JP or other wound drain Continuous IV fluids until taking adequate PO fluids	D/C Foley if not done on DOS D/C IV if taking adequate PO fluids and voiding; convert to saline loc if needed for IVPBs	D/C saline loc	N/A	N/A
Mobility/Self-Care	Total care Bed rest Turn patient q 2 h to unaffected side or back only Fracture pan Overhead trapeze	Same as Day 1	Dangle at bedside, then up in chair with assistance BID BSC/fracture pan Do not hyperflex hips; elevate affected leg when OOB PT for bedside exercises (ROM, muscle strengthening) Assist with ADLs	OOB in chair with assistance (try to ambulate from bed to chair) PT for walker ambulation and gait-training Assist with ADLs as needed PWB for ambulation BSC or elevated toilet seat	Increase ambulation in room Ambulate with assistance to bathroom (elevated toilet seat) PWB for ambulation	Ambulate in hall for short distance under supervision using PWB

Discharge Planning					
Assess for support systems and financial status	Same as Day 1	Reassess support systems and financial status	Make arrangements for discharge to home, NH, or rehab unit/facility	If discharged to home, contact home health services (nursing, PT, OT) for follow-up If discharged to rehab unit/facility, arrange for transfer	Arrange for follow-up appointment with MD if discharged to home Make final arrangements for discharge Arrange for special equipment, such as elevated toilet seat, walker, for home use if discharged to home

Clinical Pathway for Total Hip Replacement

ICD-9 Code 715.35   ELOS 6 days

Nursing Diagnosis/ Collaborative Problem	Expected Outcome (The Patient Is Expected to...)	Met/ Not Met	Reason	Date/ Initials
Pain	State that pain is relieved following appropriate interventions			
Potential for dislocation	Not experience dislocation of the operative hip			
Potential for postoperative complications (hemorrhage, infection, thromboembolitic complications)	Have Hgb and Hct WNL, stable VS, WBC WNL, and no S/S of DVT, PE, or other thromboembolitic complications			
Impaired physical mobility	Walk from room into hall using a walker with supervision; not experience complications of immobility			

Aspect of Care	Date___ Pre-admission/ Pre-op	Date___ Day 1 (DOS)	Date___ Day 2 (POD #1)	Date___ Day 3 (POD #2)	Date___ Day 4 (POD #3)	Date___ Day 5 (POD #4)	Date___ Day 6 (POD #5)
Assessment	Systems assessment Pre-op checklist Psychosocial assessment PT evaluation for assistive/ ambulatory aids; muscle strength (UE and LE)	*PACU:* Systems assessment Pain assessment VS q 15 min x 4, q 30 min x 4 NV checks with VS Check hip dressing and drain	VS and NV assessment q 4 h; check hip dressing and drain Maintain hip abduction; keep operative leg in alignment (may use knee immobilizer)	VS q 8 h with NV checks Assess for BM Assess incision for S/S of infection Maintain hip abduction/assess for dislocation Assess skin q 8 h	VS q 8 h with NV checks Assess hip incision for S/S of infection Assess LE for S/S of DVT Assess for results of laxative, if given	Same as Day 4 (POD #3)	Same as Day 5 (POD #4)

(Assessment)		Maintain hip abduction with pillow or special device (assess position) *Post-op:* Pain assessment; VS q 1 h x 4, then q 4 h with NV checks; Monitor hip dressing for drainage and drain function; Systems assessment; Check for voiding; Assess skin (especially heels) q 8 h	Assess skin (especially heels) q 8 h; Nutritional assessment, if needed; Systems assessment q 8–12 h	Same as Day 2 (POD #1)	Assess skin, especially heels QD	
Teaching	Pre-op teaching regarding surgery; pain management, post-op expectations, hip precautions; PT instruction regarding use of walker and weight-bearing expected post-op; Review plan of care/clinical pathway with patient and family	Teach/demonstrate DB & C techniques; incentive spirometer; Reinforce basic understanding of surgical procedure; Hip precautions; Teach/demonstrate procedure for ankle pumps, quad and gluteal sets	Reinforce teaching regarding hip precautions; Reinforce teaching regarding LE exercises; Teach additional pain relief measures, such as muscle relaxation and visual imagery, if appropriate; Teach purpose of anticoagulation measures	Begin discharge teaching regarding • Wound care • Pain management • Physical activity/sexual activity • Ambulation/weight-bearing exercises • Rehabilitation program complications • Meds • Hip precautions • Bleeding precautions/testing	Continue with discharge teaching	Review discharge instructions

Continued

Clinical Pathway for Total Hip Replacement *Continued*

Aspect of Care (Cont'd)	Date___ Pre-admission/ Pre-op	Date___ Day 1 (DOS)	Date___ Day 2 (POD #1)	Date___ Day 3 (POD #2)	Date___ Day 4 (POD #3)	Date___ Day 5 (POD #4)	Date___ Day 6 (POD #5)
Consults	PT for evaluation	Social worker for rehab/placement	PT for muscle strengthening exercises and post-op evaluation	PT for weight-bearing and ambulation with walker	N/A	N/A	N/A
Lab Tests	Admission labs, including CBC, SMA-6 (6/60), INR(PT)/APTT	N/A	Hgb and Hct (contact MD if Hgb ≤9 or Hct ≤28) (may be drawn DOS PM) INR(PT)/APTT	CBC and lytes INR(PT)/APTT	INR(PT)/APTT	INR(PT)/APTT	INR(PT)/APTT
Other Tests	Hip x-ray Chest x-ray ECG	Portable hip x-ray (PACU or OR)	N/A	Hip x-ray via stretcher if suspect dislocation or subluxation	N/A	N/A	N/A
Meds	Prophylactic antibiotic (cephalosporin) at least 1 h before OR Pre-anesthesia meds	Antibiotic IVPB q 6 h x 2–4 doses PCA with meperidine or morphine Antiemetic PRN Coumadin QD or heparin or Lovenex SQ q 8–12 h (contact MD for INR(PT) >3 or APTT >50) Tylenol q 4 h PRN for temp >101°F or pain Stool softener at bedtime	Same as Day 1 (DOS)	Laxative of choice if no BM Same as Day 2 (POD #1) D/C PCA; switch to IM meperidine; Percocet (Tylox) PO q 3–4 h PRN; may use Darvocet-N 100 mg	Continue with PO pain med Stool softener at bedtime Continue with Coumadin/ heparin/Lovenox per MD order based on lab Tylenol PRN for breakthrough pain or fever	Same as Day 4 (POD #3)	Same as Day 5 (POD #4)

Treatments/ Interventions	Betadine scrub (patient may do own)	I & O until IV D/C'd; Pillow or abduction pillow/splint between legs at all times while in bed; Turn patient toward unaffected side with legs abducted; TCDB q 2 h; incentive spirometer q 2 h W/A; Thigh-high antiembolism stockings; SCDs while in bed; ROM to nonoperative side; Straight cath if not voided 8 h after surgery	I & O; Keep legs abducted and turn toward unaffected side; TCDB and incentive spirometer q 2 h; Thigh-high stockings and SCDs while in bed	Dressing change and drain removal by MD; if healing, may remove dressing; Maintain abduction; Continue with pulmonary interventions; Maintain stockings	Continue with antiembolism stockings and SCDs; Assess skin, especially heels, QD; Change dressing BID or clean incision with NS; Hip precautions	Same as Day 4 (POD #3)	Same as Day 5 (POD #4)
Nutrition	NPO after 12 midnight	NPO until fully awake, then clear liquids	Full liquids → progress DAT	DAT	Same as Day 3 (POD #2)	Same as Day 4 (POD #3)	Same as Day 5 (POD #4)
Lines/Tubes/ Monitors	N/A	Continuous IV fluids; Hemovac or JP drain(s)	Same as Day 1 (DOS)	D/C IV unless vomiting or low Hgb/Hct	N/A	N/A	N/A

Continued

Clinical Pathway for Total Hip Replacement *Continued*

Aspect of Care (Cont'd)	Date_____ Pre-admission/ Pre-op	Date_____ Day 1 (DOS)	Date_____ Day 2 (POD #1)	Date_____ Day 3 (POD #2)	Date_____ Day 4 (POD #3)	Date_____ Day 5 (POD #4)	Date_____ Day 6 (POD #5)
Mobility/Self-Care	Activity ad lib	Bed rest/HOB 45° Total care Fracture pan Ankle pumps, quad and gluteal sets Overhead frame/ trapeze on bed	Dangle at bed-side, then up in chair with assistance BID using pivot technique Fracture pan/BSC Ankle pumps, quad and gluteal sets Do not hyperflex hips; elevate operative leg when OOB PT for bedside exercises, if indicated PT evaluation for special needs, such as platform walker, if not done pre-op	Up in chair with assistance 2–3 x QD BSC/elevated toilet seat Continue with exercises and hip precautions Same as Day 2 (POD #1)	Up with walker in room BID and PRN with supervision (PWB for cemented prosthesis; toe-touch for noncemented prosthesis) PT BID for progressive ambulation ROM and LE strengthening	Up with walker and into hall 3–4 x QD Continue with PT	Same as Day 5 (POD #4)
Discharge Planning	N/A	Assess home needs and sup-port; financial status	Re-assess home needs and support; collaborate with social worker about possible temporary or permanent placement and financial needs	Same as Day 2 (POD #1)	Continue to col-laborate regard-ing placement into rehab or LTC facility, as needed Involve family/ significant others in discharge planning If discharged to home, refer for home health, PT services	Same as Day 4 (POD #3)	If discharged to home, arrange for follow-up appointment as MD specified If discharged to rehab or LTC facility, commu-nicate patient information to staff

Notes

Clinical Pathway for Total Knee Replacement

ICD-9 Code 715.36   ELOS 6 days

Nursing Diagnosis/Collaborative Problem	Expected Outcome (The Patient Is Expected to...)	Met/Not Met	Reason	Date/Initials
Pain	State that pain is relieved following appropriate interventions			
Impaired physical mobility	Walk from room into hall using a walker with supervision; not experience complications of immobility			
Potential for postoperative complications (hemorrhage, infection, thromboembolitic problems)	Have Hgb and Hct WNL, stable VS, WBC WNL, and no S/S of DVT, PE, or other thromboembolitic complications			

Aspect of Care	Date ___ Pre-admission/ Pre-op	Date ___ Day 1 (DOS)	Date ___ Day 2 (POD #1)	Date ___ Day 3 (POD #2)	Date ___ Day 4 (POD #3)	Date ___ Day 5 (POD #4)	Date ___ Day 6 (POD #5)
Assessment	Systems assessment Pre-op checklist Psychosocial assessment PT evaluation for assistive/ambulatory aids; muscle strength	*PACU:* Systems assessment Pain assessment VS q 15 min x 4, q 30 min x 4 NV checks with VS Check knee dressing for drainage; check drain	VS and NV assessment q 4 h; check knee dressing and drain Maintain knee immobilizer Assess skin q 8 h Systems assessment q 8–12 h	VS q 8 h with NV checks Assess for BM Assess incision for S/S of infection Assess skin q 8 h Systems assessment	VS q 8 h with NV checks Assess knee incision for S/S of infection Assess LE for S/S of DVT Assess for results of laxative, if given Assess skin, especially heels QD	Same as Day 4 (POD #3)	Same as Day 5 (POD #4)

Maintain knee immobilizer, if ordered *Post-op:* Pain assessment VS q 1 h x 4, then q 4 h NV checks with VS Check knee dressing for drainage (with VS) Maintain knee immobilizer, if ordered Systems assessment Assess skin (especially heels) q 8 h Check for voiding						
Teaching	Pre-op teaching regarding surgery, pain management, post-op expectations, CPM machine Review plan of care/clinical pathway with patient and family	*Pre-op:* Reinforce pre-op teaching regarding surgery, pain management, post-op expectations PT instruction regarding use of walker and weight-bearing expected post-op	Reinforce teaching regarding LE exercises Teach purpose and use of CPM machine Teach additional pain relief measures, such as muscle relaxation and visual imagery, if appropriate	Reinforce information on CPM machine and exercises	Begin discharge teaching regarding • Wound care • Pain management • Physical activity/sexual activity • Ambulation/weight bearing • Exercises • Rehabilitation program	Continue with discharge teaching
						Review discharge instructions

Continued

Clinical Pathway for Total Knee Replacement *Continued*

Aspect of Care (Cont'd)	Date ___ Pre-admission/	Date ___ Day 1 (DOS)	Date ___ Day 2 (POD #1)	Date ___ Day 3 (POD #2)	Date ___ Day 4 (POD #3)	Date ___ Day 5 (POD #4)	Date ___ Day 6 (POD #5)
Teaching (Cont'd)	PT instruction regarding use of walker and weight-bearing expected post-op	*Post-op:* Teach/demonstrate procedure for DB & C and incentive spirometer Reinforce basic understanding of surgical procedure Teach/demonstrate procedure for ankle pumps, quad sets, and gluteal sets			• Complications • Meds • Use of CPM after discharge, if indicated • Bleeding precautions/testing		
Consults	PT for evaluation	Social worker for rehab/placement	PT for muscle strengthening exercises and post-op evaluation	PT for weight-bearing and ambulation with walker	N/A	N/A	N/A
Lab Tests	Admission labs, including CBC, SMA-6 (6/60), and INR(PT)/APTT	N/A	Hgb and Hct (contact MD if Hgb ≤9 or Hct ≤28) (may be drawn DOS PM) INR(PT)/APTT	CBC and lytes Same as Day 2 (POD #1)	INR(PT)/APTT	INR(PT)/APTT	INR(PT)/APTT
Other Tests	Knee x-ray Chest x-ray ECG	Portable knee x-ray (PACU or OR)	N/A	N/A	N/A	N/A	N/A

CLINICAL PATHWAY FOR TOTAL KNEE REPLACEMENT **135**

			Same as Day 1 (DOS)			Same as Day 4 (POD #3)	Same as Day 5 (POD #4)
Meds	Prophylactic antibiotic (cephalosporin) at least 1 h before OR Pre-anesthesia meds	Antibiotic IVPB q 6 h x 2–4 doses PCA with meperidine or morphine Antiemetic PRN Coumadin QD or heparin or Lovenox SQ q 8–12 h (contact MD for INR(PT) >3 or APTT >50) Tylenol q 4 h PRN for temp >101°F or pain Stool softener at bedtime	Same as Day 1 (DOS)	Laxative of choice if no BM Same as Day 2 (POD #1) D/C PCA; switch to IM meperidine; Percocet (Tylox) PO q 3–4 h PRN; may use Darvocet-N 100 mg	Continue with PO pain med Stool softener at bedtime Continue with Coumadin/heparin/Lovenox per MD order based on INR(PT)/APTT Tylenol PRN for breakthrough pain or fever	Same as Day 4 (POD #3)	Same as Day 5 (POD #4)
Treatments/ Interventions	Betadine scrub (patient may do own)	I & O until IVs D/C'd Elevate surgical leg on pillow Thigh-high antiembolism stockings SCDs while in bed TCDB q 2 h; incentive spirometer q 2 h W/A ROM to non-operative side Straight cath if not voided 8 h after surgery	I & O Elevate surgical leg Continue antiembolism stockings and SCDs while in bed TCDB and incentive spirometer q 2 h W/A	Dressing change and drain removal by MD; if healing, may remove dressing Continue with pulmonary interventions CPM machine to surgical leg 4–8 h QD per MD order; use knee immobilizer when not in CPM machine (may be started POD #1)	Continue with antiembolism stockings and SCDs Increase ROM on CPM machine as MD specified Assess skin, especially heel QD Change dressing BID; clean incision with NS	Same as Day 4 (POD #3)	Same as Day 5 (POD #4)

Continued

Clinical Pathway for Total Knee Replacement *Continued*

Aspect of Care (Cont'd)	Date_____ Pre-admission/ Pre-op	Date_____ Day 1 (DOS)	Date_____ Day 2 (POD #1)	Date_____ Day 3 (POD #2)	Date_____ Day 4 (POD #3)	Date_____ Day 5 (POD #4)	Date_____ Day 6 (POD #5)
Nutrition	NPO after 12 midnight	NPO until fully awake, then clear liquids	Full liquids; progress DAT	DAT	Same as Day 3 (POD #2)	Same as Day 4 (POD #3)	Same as Day 5 (POD #4)
Lines/Tubes/ Monitors	IV with 18g cath	Continuous IV fluids Hemovac or JP drain(s)	Same as Day 1 (DOS)	D/C IV unless vomiting or low Hgb and Hct	N/A	N/A	N/A
Mobility/Self-Care	N/A	Bed rest Total care Fracture pan Ankle pumps, quad and gluteal sets (10 x) q 2 h Overhead frame/ trapeze on bed	Dangle at bedside, then up in chair with assistance BID using pivot technique (elevate leg in chair) PT for bedside exercises, if indicated PT evaluation for special needs, such as platform walker, if not done pre-op	Up in chair with assistance 2–3 x QD Elevated toilet seat/BSC PT for beginning ambulation, ROM, and LE strengthening exercises; PWB (unless non-cemented prosthesis; toe touch for noncemented prosthesis)	Up with walker in room BID and PRN with supervision (PWB for cemented prosthesis; toe-touch for noncemented prosthesis) PT BID for progressive ambulation, ROM, and LE strengthening	Up with walker in room and into hall 3–4 x QD Continue with PT	Same as Day 5 (POD #4)
Discharge Planning	N/A	Assess home needs and support; financial status	Re-assess home needs and support; work with social worker on possible temporary or permanent placement	Same as Day 2 (POD #1)	Continue to collaborate regarding placement into rehab or LTC facility, as needed Involve family/ significant others in discharge planning If discharged to home, refer to home health, PT services	Same as Day 4 (POD #3)	If discharged to home, arrange for follow-up appointment as MD specified If discharged to rehab or LTC facility, communicate patient information to staff at post-hospital facility

Notes

Clinical Pathway for Lower Extremity Amputation (Nontraumatic, Elective)

ICD-9 Code 785.4/84.15   ELOS 5 days

Nursing Diagnosis/ Collaborative Problem	Expected Outcome (The Patient Is Expected to...)	Met/ Not Met	Reason	Date/ Initials
Pain	State that pain is relieved or controlled following appropriate interventions			
Potential for postoperative complications (hemorrhage, wound or bone infection, ischemia, pneumonia)	Have Hgb and Hct WNL, stable VS, WBC WNL, incision clean and dry, palpable and equal LE pulses, clear breath sounds			
Impaired physical mobility	Transfer from bed to wheelchair independently; ambulation with walker independently			
Potential for ineffective coping/body image disturbance	Participate in self-care; ventilate feelings about impact of surgery; identify personal support systems			

Aspect of Care	Date _____ Pre-admission/ Pre-op	Date _____ Day 1 (DOS)	Date _____ Day 2 (POD #1)	Date _____ Day 3 (POD #2)	Date _____ Day 4 (POD #3)	Date _____ Day 5 (POD #4)
Assessment	Pre-op checklist Systems assessment Psychosocial assessment	*PACU:* Systems assessment Pain assessment VS q 15 min x 4, then q 30 min x 4 Circulation checks with VS Check stump dressing for increasing drainage Assess output from JP or other wound drain, if present *Post-op:* Systems/pain assessment VS q 1 h x 4, then q 4 h, if stable Circulation checks with VS Check stump dressing for increasing drainage Measure drainage from wound drain q 8 h Check for voiding	VS and circulation checks QID (assess operative and nonoperative sides) Check stump dressing and wound drain, if present Systems assessment with focus on breath and bowel sounds Skin assessment, especially heel	VS and circulation checks QID FSBS if diabetic Systems assessment with focus on breath sounds and skin, especially heel and other pressure points Monitor incision for S/S of infection during dressing changes Assess for BM	VS and circulation checks q 8 h Monitor incision for S/S of infection during dressing changes Systems assessment with focus on skin FSBS if diabetic Assess for BM	Same as Day 4

Clinical Pathway for Lower Extremity Amputation (Nontraumatic, Elective) *Continued*

Aspect of Care (Cont'd)	Date _____ Pre-admission/ Pre-op	Date _____ Day 1 (DOS)	Date _____ Day 2 (POD #1)	Date _____ Day 3 (POD #2)	Date _____ Day 4 (POD #3)	Date _____ Day 5 (POD #4)
Teaching	Reinforce pre-op teaching regarding • Surgical procedure • Incision/dressing • Pain management (including phantom limb pain) • Post-op care expectations / Review clinical path/plan of care with patient and family / Visit by amputee support volunteer (if possible pre-op)	Teach/demonstrate procedure for DB & C, incentive spirometer / Reinforce basic understanding of surgical procedure / Orient to hospital and unit / Teach additional pain relief measures, such as muscle relaxation and visual imagery, if patient is not cognitively impaired	Same as Day 1 / Visit by amputee support volunteer, if not done pre-op	Begin discharge teaching with patient and family regarding • Wound care • Pain management/phantom limb pain • Rehab program, if candidate • Meds • Complications / Reinforce ROM and muscle strengthening exercises for UE and LE	Review discharge instructions as per Day 3 / Provide written materials on amputation recovery / Start teaching patient to wrap stump with compressive ace wrap, if no active drainage from stump / Review ROM and muscle strengthening exercises	Same as Day 4
Consults	PT/OT for evaluation of UE and LE function / Evaluation for prosthesis	Respiratory therapy, if available, for pulmonary evaluation	PT/OT if not obtained pre-op / Dietician if patient has diabetes or hyperlipidemia/ hypercholesterolemia	N/A	N/A	N/A
Lab Tests	Admission labs, including CBC, SMA-6 (6/60), INR(PT)/APTT, lipid profile	Hgb and Hct, lytes, glucose, if diabetic	Daily FBS if diabetic	Same as Day 2	Same as Day 3	Same as Day 4

Other Tests	Chest x-ray and ECG if >40 years old or history of cardiac disease Arterial flow studies Ankle/brachial index evaluation	N/A	N/A	N/A	N/A	N/A
Meds	Prophylactic antibiotic at least 1 h before OR Pre-anesthesia meds	PCA or IM meperidine or morphine Toradol IM for breakthrough pain PRN Antibiotic (cephalosporin) IVPB q 6–8 h x 3–4 doses Antiemetic PRN Regular insulin coverage if diabetic Tylenol supp PRN for ↑ temp Stool softener at bedtime	D/C PCA; switch to IM or PO opioid such as Percocet (Tylox) PO q 3–4 h 1–2 tabs Tylenol 2 tabs q 3–4 h PRN Insulin coverage, if diabetic Antispasmodic, anticonvulsant, or beta blocker for phantom limb pain Stool softener	Oral opioid Insulin coverage, if diabetic Laxative PRN Meds for phantom limb pain Stool softener	Same as Day 3	Same as Day 4
Treatments/ Interventions	N/A	Knee immobilizer, if ordered by surgeon for extension/ protection I & O until IV fluids D/C'd	Knee immobilizer, if ordered Reinforce stump dressing DB & C q 2 h W/A	MD to change dressing or remove dressing and drain Bed cradle Dressing change BID; clean incision with NS and secure with noncompressive ace wrap	When no active drainage, use compressive ace wrap (figure–8) Clean incision BID with NS Interventions for phantom limb pain	Same as Day 4

Continued

Clinical Pathway for Lower Extremity Amputation (Nontraumatic, Elective) *Continued*

Aspect of Care (Cont'd)	Date ____ Pre-admission/ Pre-op	Date ____ Day 1 (DOS)	Date ____ Day 2 (POD #1)	Date ____ Day 3 (POD #2)	Date ____ Day 4 (POD #3)	Date ____ Day 5 (POD #4)
Treatment/ Interventions (Cont'd)		Reinforce stump dressing PRN and secure with noncompressive ace wrap	Respiratory therapy treatments (incentive spirometer, nebulizer as needed)	Provide emotional support		
		Provide emotional support	Provide emotional support	Nonpharmacologic interventions for relief of phantom limb pain, if present		
		Keep stump elevated on pillow for no more than 24 h	Bed cradle			
		Heel protector/pillow for nonoperative leg	Evaluation for nonpharmacologic pain relief measures for phantom limb pain (e.g., TENS, distraction, ultrasound)			
		TCDB q 2 h				
		Bed cradle				
Nutrition	NPO after 12 midnight	Clear → full liquids as tolerated	Full liquids → DAT (may need diabetic or fat-restricted diet)	DAT (unless diabetic or need fat restriction)	Same as Day 3	Same as Day 4
Lines/Tubes/ Monitors	N/A	Foley cath to straight drainage during OR *PACU:* Continuous IV infusion of Lactated Ringer's or 5% D/½NS *Post-op:* Continuous IV fluids (dextrose may not be ordered if patient is diabetic)	D/C IV when taking adequate fluids; convert to saline loc if needed for IV antibiotics	N/A	N/A	N/A

Mobility/Self-Care	Activity ad lib	Monitor output from wound and drain, if present Bed rest Assist with ADLs as needed Turn q 2 h with assistance; support stump Overhead trapeze	Bedside PT for ROM and muscle strengthening exercises OOB in chair BID Prevent prolonged hip flexion Overhead trapeze	Stand at bedside Transfer to chair BID using walker BSC Overhead trapeze Prone-lying TID for 20–30 min, if tolerated	PT for walker ambulation and gait training; ROM and muscle strengthening education OT, if needed, for ADLs retraining Walk to bathroom using walker Encourage prone-lying Overhead trapeze	Same as Day 4
Discharge Planning	N/A	Assess for home situation, support systems, and financial status	Contact rehab unit or hospital if potential for rehabilitation If not rehab candidate, social worker to evaluate for placement in home with home health services support or NH placement	Continue to arrange for discharge to NH, home, or rehab facility Assess financial needs and support systems	Make final arrangements for placement	Transfer to rehab unit/facility, if candidate Discharge to home with support from home health or discharge to NH (may use nursing, PT/OT in home) Arrange for follow-up in amputee or other appropriate clinic as outpatient or arrange for follow-up appointment with MD as specified

Unit

V

Problems of Urinary Elimination/ Renal and Urologic Health Problems

Clinical Pathway for Acute Renal Failure: Medical Management

ICD-9 Code 316   ELOS 5 days

Nursing Diagnosis/ Collaborative Problem	Expected Outcome (The Patient Is Expected to...)	Met/ Not Met	Reason	Date/ Initials
Altered renal tissue perfusion	Have a return of usual renal function with stable renal function tests			
Fluid volume deficit or excess	Have adequate urinary output and no indications of dehydration or edema			
Altered nutritional status	Understand rationale for dietary restrictions and follow recommended diet			
Fatigue	Perform ADLs independently			
High risk for infection	Exhibit no signs or symptoms of infection			

Aspect of Care	Date____ Day 1	Date____ Day 2	Date____ Day 3	Date____ Day 4	Date____ Day 5
Assessment	Systems assessment q shift with particular attention to renal • Decreased urine volume, frequency, change in color, odor VS and NS q 4 h Assess for underlying cause	Same as Day 1 Monitor closely for renal failure progression, uremia Assess need for dialysis (severe acidosis and/or hyperkalemia)	Same as Day 2	Same as Day 3 VS and NS q 8 h	Same as Day 4

Assess for Chvostek's or Trousseau's sign, neck vein distention, cap refill Monitor med levels; assess need to adjust med (e.g., those excreted or metabolized in kidney) Monitor for complications • Acidosis, hyperkalemia • Hypertension, overload • Infection, uremia, ileus • Pneumonia, GI bleed Psychosocial assessment				
Teaching	Orient to hospital and unit Prepare for diagnostic tests Provide information about diagnosis Involve family in care of patient as appropriate Review plan of care/clinical pathway with patient and family	Continue to provide information regarding diagnosis and diagnostic tests Explain dialysis, if needed	Diet education and fluid restriction Meds: action, side effects, time Importance of rest and gradually increasing activity	Same as Day 3 Instruct in S/S of renal failure, infection Based on identified cause of renal failure, provide prevention or management information	Review meds, diet, lab work, fluid and activity restriction Instruct to do daily wts using same scale Instruct in S/S of renal failure, infection

Continued

Clinical Pathway for Acute Renal Failure: Medical Management Continued

Aspect of Care (Cont'd)	Date____ Day 1	Date____ Day 2	Date____ Day 3	Date____ Day 4	Date____ Day 5
Consults	Dietician Nephrologist Social worker	N/A	N/A	N/A	N/A
Lab Tests	Lytes, BUN, CR, Mg^{+2}, phosphorus, bicarb, calcium, protein, albumin, lipids CBC with diff INR(PT)/APTT Urine for: C & S, Cr, osmolality, lytes	Lytes, BUN, Cr Hct and Hgb	Same as Day 2	Lytes, BUN, Cr, Hgb and Hct, Mg^{+2}, phosphorus, albumin, protein	Serum: BUN, Cr, lytes Urine: U/A, lytes, osmolality
Other Tests	Chest and KUB x-ray CT scan with contrast Renal sonogram, ECG	Aortorenal angiography Possible cystoscopy or retrograde pyelography	Possible renal biopsy	N/A	N/A
Meds	*Acidosis and/or hyperkalemia:* • Kayexalate followed by sorbitol • If K+ >6.5 mEq give 50% glucose and regular insulin • Sodium bicarb citrate or calcium gluconate	Antihypertensive Cardiotonic Diuretic Vitamin and mineral supplement Stool softener	Same as Day 2	Antihypertensive	Same as Day 4

Treatments/ Interventions				
Anithypertensives: • Hydralazine • Methyldopa • Propranolol Cardiotonic such as digoxin Hyperphosphatemia: • Calcium carbonate or other phosphate binders Vitamins and minerals (vitamin D, folic acid) Stool softener Strict I & O measure of all body fluid output Urine specific gravity each void Daily wts Frequent skin and oral care O$_2$ per NC, if needed Safety precautions Incentive spirometer q 2 h W/A Strict aseptic techniques for all procedures Guaiac all stools	Same as Day 1	Same as Day 2	Strict I & O Daily wts Skin and mouth care	Same as Day 4

Continued

Clinical Pathway for Acute Renal Failure: Medical Management *Continued*

Aspect of Care (Cont'd)	Date _____ Day 1	Date _____ Day 2	Date _____ Day 3	Date _____ Day 4	Date _____ Day 5
Nutrition	High fat and carbohydrate, low protein diet with NA+ and K+ restriction Fluid restriction based on lytes	Same as Day 1	Same as Day 2	Same as Day 3	Same as Day 4
Lines/Tubes/Monitors	IV fluids (depends on phase)	Same as Day 1	Convert IV to saline loc	Saline loc	D/C saline loc
Mobility/Self-Care	Bed rest ROM q 4 h W/A Prevent complications of immobility	OOB as tolerated ROM	OOB as tolerated Ambulate in room as tolerated	OOB and ambulate as tolerated	OOB and ambulate as tolerated
Discharge Planning	Social worker to assess need for social services, financial status, health insurance and coverage, home environment, need for placement and family support	Same as Day 1	Assess ability to perform ADLS, home environment, and need for assistive/adaptive devices	Arrange for outpatient blood and urine tests Ensure transportation available Verify ability to pay for meds and lab work Continue ADL assessment Refer to home health	Continue as Day 4 Arrange for follow-up visit with MD

Notes

Clinical Pathway for Acute Renal Failure: Peritoneal Dialysis (PD)

ICD-9 Code 316   ELOS 5 days

Nursing Diagnosis/ Collaborative Problem	Expected Outcome (The Patient Is Expected to...)	Met/ Not Met	Reason	Date/ Initials
Altered renal tissue perfusion	Have stable renal function			
Fluid volume excess (fluid accumulation)	Maintain ideal body weight for age, height, and body build			
Fluid volume deficit (rapid removal of fluid during PD treatment)	Have no signs or symptoms of dehydration			
Altered nutritional status	Understand and follow recommended diet and fluid intake			
Fatigue	Perform ADLs independently and return to usual day-to-day activities			
High risk for infection	Exhibit no signs or symptoms of infection			

Aspect of Care	Date____ Day 1	Date____ Day 2	Date____ Day 3	Date____ Day 4	Date____ Day 5
Assessment	Systems assessment with attention to renal VS and neuro signs q 4 h Assess for underlying cause Assess for neck vein distention, cap refill	Same as Day 1	Same as Day 2	Same as Day 3 VS and NS q 8 h	Same as Day 4

Observe for indications of cath obstruction, displacement, kinking, obstruction Monitor for infection, anorexia, uremia, dyspnea Check PD dressing for drainage Monitor med levels; assess need to adjust meds, e.g., those excreted or metabolized in kidney Monitor for complications • Peritonitis, leakage and extravasation of dialysate, hyperglycemia, hypoproteinemia, wt gain Psychosocial assessment				
Teaching	Orient to hospital and unit Prepare for diagnostic tests Provide information about diagnosis Instruct regarding need for PD, cath insertion procedure,	Continue to provide information regarding diagnosis and treatment	Diet education and fluid restiction Meds: action, side effects, time Importance of rest and gradually increasing activity	Continue diet and med teaching Reinforce importance of rest and gradually increasing activity Home PD instruction if needed	Same as Day 4

Continued

Clinical Pathway for Acute Renal Failure: Peritoneal Dialysis (PD) *Continued*

Aspect of Care (Cont'd)	Date___ Day 1	Date___ Day 2	Date___ Day 3	Date___ Day 4	Date___ Day 5
Teaching *(Cont'd)*	and how it is performed Involve family in care of patient as appropriate Review plan of care/clinical pathway with patient and family				
Consults	Dietician Nephrologist Social worker	N/A	N/A	N/A	N/A
Lab Tests	*Admission:* Lytes, BUN, Cr, Mg^{+2}, phosphorus, bicarb, calcium, protein, albumin, lipids CBC with diff Urine for C & S, Cr, osmolality, lytes Peritoneal fluid for cell count, C & S *Post PD:* Lytes, BUN and Cr	Lytes, BUN, Cr Protein, CBC Peritoneal fluid for cell count	Same as Day 2	Lytes, Bun, Cr Peritoneal fluid for cell count	Lytes, BUN, Cr Protein, CBC Peritoneal fluid for cell count
Other Tests	Chest and KUB x-ray CT scan with contrast Renal sonogram, ECG	N/A	N/A	N/A	N/A

Meds	Stool softener Heparin, KCl to dialysate Antibiotics if peritonitis suspected (do not add KCl) Other meds • Home meds • Dependent on cause	Same as Day 1	Same as Day 2	Same as Day 3	Same as Day 4
Treatments/ Interventions	Strict I & O measure of all body fluid output Daily wts Frequent skin and oral care Safety precautions Aseptic technique for procedures PD procedure • VS before, during, and after • Measure abdominal girth • Warm/room temp dialysate • I & O • Monitor for respiratory distress and pain • Record inflow, dwell, and outflow times	Same as Day 1	Same as Day 2	Same as Day 3	Same as Day 4

Continued

Aspect of Care (Cont'd)	Date ___ Day 1	Date ___ Day 2	Date ___ Day 3	Date ___ Day 4	Date ___ Day 5
Treatments/ Interventions (Cont'd)	• Sterile technique • Dressing and tubing change QD				
Nutrition	Protein intake to 1.2–5 kg/day, low Na$^+$ and K$^+$ Fluid restriction to 1 L/day	Same as Day 1	Same as Day 2	Same as Day 3	Same as Day 4
Lines/Tubes/ Monitors	IV to saline loc	Same as Day 1	Same as Day 2	Same as Day 3	D/C saline loc
Mobility/Self-Care	Bed rest with BRPs ROM q 4 h W/A Prevent complications of immobility	OOB to chair as tolerated	OOB and ambulate as tolerated	Same as Day 3	Same as Day 4
Discharge Planning	Assess need for social services, financial status, health insurance and coverage, home environment, need for placement, and family support	Same as Day 1	Assess ability to perform ADLs, home environment, and need for assistive/ adaptive devices	Assess ability to perform ADLs Identify any need for changes in the home and assistive/adaptive devices Refer to home health nurse	Continue as Day 4 Arrange for follow-up appointment with MD

Notes

Clinical Pathway for Nephrectomy

ICD-9 Code **593.2/55.51**   ELOS **5 days**

Nursing Diagnosis/Collaborative Problem	Expected Outcome (The Patient Is Expected to...)	Met/Not Met	Reason	Date/Initials
Impaired skin integrity	Have a healed incision			
Pain	State pain is relieved or controlled with PO medication			
High risk for fluid volume deficit	Eat a balanced diet with a fluid intake of 1500–2000 mL per day and no indications of dehydration			
High risk for infection	Have a normal WBC count and be afebrile			

Aspect of Care	Date ___ Pre-admission/Pre-op	Date ___ Day 1 (DOS)	Date ___ Day 2 (POD #1)	Date ___ Day 3 (POD #2)	Date ___ Day 4 (POD #3)	Date ___ Day 5 (POD# 5)
Assessment	Systems assessment Pre-op check list Psychosocial assessment	*PACU:* Systems and pain assessment VS q 15 min x 4, then q 30 min x 2 Check dressing for drainage Ensure all drains/tubes patent *Post-op:* Systems assessment	System and pain assessment VS q 4 h Inspect incision site for bleeding, drainage, redness, edema Monitor for infection, hemorrhage, pneumothorax	Same as Day 2	System and pain assessment VS q 4 h Monitor wound for infection, drainage	Same as Day 4 VS q 8 h

(Assessment)		VS q 1 h x 4, then q 4 h; Monitor for hemorrhage, pneumothorax, volume deficit; Observe color, consistency, amt of output from drainage tubes				
Teaching	Orient to hospital and unit; Reinforce information about surgery • Location of incision • Tubes and drains • Post-op care • TCDB • Leg exercises • Pain management; Involve family in care of patient as appropriate; Review plan of care/clinical pathway with patient and family	Reinforce information on ROM and incentive spirometry	Provide information on • S/S of infection, urinary tract infection • Need to gradually increase activity to avoid fatigue • Need for rest periods	Same as Day 2; Inform patient not to take over-the-counter meds without checking with MD	Explain how to prevent additional renal problems; Reinforce previous information	Same as Day 4
Consults	Anesthesia and medical clearance for surgery; Social services	N/A	N/A	N/A	N/A	N/A

Continued

Clinical Pathway for Nephrectomy *Continued*

Aspect of Care (Cont'd)	Date ___ Pre-admission/ Pre-op	Date ___ Day 1 (DOS)	Date ___ Day 2 (POD #1)	Date ___ Day 3 (POD #2)	Date ___ Day 4 (POD #3)	Date ___ Day 5 (POD #4)
Lab Tests	CBC with diff, lytes, BUN, Cr, INR(PT)/APTT, Type and screen U/A	Hgb and Hct	Lytes, BUN, Cr Hct and Hgb	Same as Day 2	Hgb and Hct, lytes, BUN, Cr	N/A
Other Tests	Chest x-ray ECG KUB	N/A	N/A	N/A	N/A	N/A
Meds	IV antibiotics before surgery	Pain meds via PCA pump or IM IV antibiotics x 48 h	Same as Day 1	D/C PCA pump PO analgesia D/C antibiotics	Same as Day 3	Same as Day 4
Treatments/ Interventions	Wt Thigh-high anti-embolism stockings	Prevent drains/tubes from obstruction, kinking; position to avoid tension on suture line Strict I & O Daily wts Thigh-high anti-embolism stockings and SCDs TCDB q 2 h Incentive spirometer q 2 h W/A Strict aseptic techniques	Same as Day 1	Same as Day 2 D/C SCDs	I & O Daily wts Incentive spirometer q 4 h W/A Thigh-high anti-embolism stockings	Same as Day 4

Nutrition	NPO after 12 midnight	NPO until bowel sounds present, then clear liquids	Clear liquids; advance as tolerated	DAT Low Na$^+$	Same as Day 3	Same as Day 4
Lines/Tubes/Monitors	N/A	Continuous IV fluids Observe amt, color, and consistency of drainage from all tubes Foley cath	Same as Day 1 Remove Foley cath	Convert IV to saline loc All drains and tubes removed	D/C saline loc	N/A
Mobility/Self-Care	Activity as tolerated	Bed rest ROM q 4 h W/A Prevent complications of immobility	OOB to chair as tolerated ROM q 4 h	OOB to chair as tolerated Ambulate as tolerated ROM q shift Prevent complications of immobility	OOB and ambulate in hall as tolerated	Same as Day 4
Discharge Planning	N/A	Assess need for social services, financial status, health insurance and coverage, home environment, need for placement, and family support	Same as Day 1	Assess ability to perform ADLs, home environment, and need for assistive/adaptive devices	Refer to home health	Arrange for follow-up appointment with MD

Clinical Pathway for Transurethral Resection of the Prostate (TURP)

Nursing Diagnosis/ Collaborative Problem	Expected Outcome (The Patient Is Expected to...)	Met/ Not Met	Reason	Date/ Initials
Potential for altered pattern of urinary elimination: retention	Have normal flow of clear urine			
High risk for hemorrhage	Have Hgb and Hct within normal limits and void clear, yellow urine			
Pain	State that pain is relieved and bladder spasms are managed with medication			

Aspect of Care	Date___ Pre-admission/Pre-op	Date___ Day 1 (DOS)	Date___ Day 2 (POD #1)	Date___ Day 3 (POD #2)
Assessment	Systems assessment Pre-op check list Psychosocial assessment	*PACU:* VS q 15 min x 4, then q 30 min x 4 Systems and pain assessment Check Foley for drainage and hematuria *Post-op:* Systems and pain assessment Check Foley for drainage, hematuria, obstruction	Systems assessment q shift VS q 4 h Monitor for signs of cath obstruction, complications Assess for pain, bladder spasm Assess for spontaneous voiding	VS q 8 h Continue to monitor for complications and pain

Teaching	Orient to hospital and unit Teach regarding Foley cath, leg exercises, type of anesthesia, methods of pain relief Review plan of care/clinical pathway with patient and family	Check Foley position (taped to abdomen or thigh) Monitor for complications • Hemorrhage • Hyponatremia • Bladder perforation Involve family in care of patient as appropriate Leg exercises to prevent DVT	Teach patient how to do Kegel exercises Teach signs and symptoms of UTI Instruct patient to avoid strenuous exercises for 2–3 wks q surgery Explain that slight hematuria may occur for up to 2 wks	Instruct patient to call MD if pain becomes severe, gross hematuria occurs, or if unable to void
Consults	Medical clearance for surgery	N/A	N/A	N/A
Lab Tests	CBC, lytes Acid phosphatase Type and screen U/A, INR(PT)/APTT	N/A	Hgb and Hct	N/A
Other Tests	Chest x-ray ECG	N/A	N/A	N/A
Meds	Prophylactic antibiotics before OR	Analgesics (meperidine, acetaminophen) q 4 h	PO analgesic Continue antispasmodics if needed	Continue as Day 2

Continued

Clinical Pathway for Transurethral Resection of the Prostate (TURP) *Continued*

Aspect of Care (Cont'd)	Date_____ Pre-admission/Pre-op	Date_____ Day 1 (DOS)	Date_____ Day 2 (POD #1)	Date_____ Day 3 (POD #2)
Meds (Cont'd)		Antispasmodic (dicyclomine hydrochloride or oxybutynin)		
Treatments/ Interventions	Thigh-high antiembolism stockings Emotional support Encourage to ventilate feeling about surgical procedure	*PACU:* Irrigate Foley cath if needed *Post-op:* Thigh-high antiembolism stockings and SCDs Irrigate Foley, if needed Strict I & O	Thigh-high antiembolism stockings I & O Remove Foley Progressive urine collection	Thigh-high antiembolism stockings I & O
Nutrition	NPO after 12 midnight	NPO until fully awake, then clear liquids	DAT Encourage fluids to 2 L/day Caffeine and spicy food in moderation	Same as Day 2
Lines/Tubes/Monitors	N/A	Continuous IV fluids Foley cath to straight drainage CBI with NS or other MD specified fluid to keep urine clear	D/C IV D/C Foley cath and CBI	N/A
Mobility/Self-Care	N/A	*Epidural anesthesia:* Flat in bed x 8 h, then increase HOB	OOB and ambulate as tolerated	Same as Day 2

	General anesthesia: OOB to chair as tolerated Bed rest if CBI	Same as Day 1	Refer to home health as needed Arrange for follow-up visit with MD
Discharge Planning	N/A	Determine if supplies needed at home Assess family support at home to assist with ADLs and other care needs after discharge	

Unit
VI

Problems of Digestion and Elimination/ Gastrointestinal Health Problems

▼ ▼ ▼

Clinical Pathway for GI Bleeding (Nonvariceal)

ICD-9 Code 578.9   ELOS 4 days

Nursing Diagnosis/Collaborative Problem	Expected Outcome (The Patient Is Expected to...)	Met/Not Met	Reason	Date/Initials
Fluid volume deficit (hypovolemia)	Have stable VS and no evidence of active bleeding			
Electrolyte imbalance	Have lytes WNL and no S/S of electrolyte imbalance			
Potential for recurrent GI bleed	Follow discharge instructions regarding meds, diet, lifestyle changes, early detection			

Aspect of Care	Date ___ Day 1	Date ___ Day 2	Date ___ Day 3	Date ___ Day 4
Assessment	VS q 1 → 4 h, depending on stability Monitor vomitus and stool for gross and occult blood Systems assessment	VS q 2 → 4 h, depending on stability Monitor vomitus and stool Systems assessment Assess for weakness, postural hypotension	VS QID Monitor vomitus and stool Systems assessment Assess for weakness, postural hypotension	VS QID Systems assessment Monitor stools for OB
Teaching	Orient to hospital and unit Review clinical pathway/plan of care with patient and family Reinforce importance of NPO, meds, IVs, and diagnostic studies	Teach pre- and post-test care for endoscopic examination	Begin discharge teaching including • Meds • Diet • Lifestyle changes • When to call MD • Monitoring stools	Reinforce/review discharge instructions

Consults	Gastroenterology/surgery Social worker	N/A	Dietician	N/A
Lab Tests	CBC with diff, SMA-6 (6/60), INR(PT)/APTT, type and crossmatch, stools for OB	Hgb and Hct, stools for OB	Hgb and Hct, stools for OB	Hgb and Hct
Other Tests	Chest X-ray if >40 years old or if history of cardiac disease	Endoscopy	N/A	N/A
Meds	Zantac or other H_2 blocker continuous IV or IVPB Blood transfusions until Hgb and Hct increase to baseline range D/C all other nonessential meds	Same as Day 1 (blood, if indicated for low Hgb and Hct)	PO antacids, carafate, and/or H_2 blocker D/C IV meds	PO antacids, Carafate, and/or H_2 blocker
Treatments/ Interventions	I & O q 8 h HOB elevated at least 30° unless severely hypotensive If severely hypotensive, may need shock blocks Provide emotional support	Same as Day 1	D/C I & O	N/A
Nutrition	NPO	NPO or clear liquids	Clear → full liquids; advance DAT (may need special diet if peptic ulcer disease, diverticulitis, or inflammatory bowel disease	DAT (or special diet for peptic ulcer disease, diverticulitis, inflammatory bowel disease)

Continued

Clinical Pathway for GI Bleeding (Nonvariceal) Continued

Aspect of Care (Cont'd)	Date____ Day 1	Date____ Day 2	Date____ Day 3	Date____ Day 4
Lines/Tubes/Monitors	Continuous IV fluids with KCl for volume, lyte replacement (18g) If upper GI bleeding, may use NGT to low suction	Continue with IV fluids May clamp or D/C NGT if bleeding subsides	D/C NGT if still present D/C IV and convert to saline loc	D/C saline loc, if present
Mobility/Self-Care	Bed rest Assist with ADLs as needed	Bed rest Assist with ADLs as needed	BSC or BRPs with supervision Assist with ADLs as needed	Up ad lib
Discharge Planning	Assess support systems and financial needs; assess need for home health services or NH placement	Same as Day 1	Complete arrangements for home health or NH placement Arrange for follow-up appointment with MD as specified	Discharge to home or NH Follow-up appointment with MD or clinic

Notes

Clinical Pathway for Colon Resection (Without Ostomy)

ICD-9 Code **562.10/45.79**   ELOS **6 days**

Nursing Diagnosis/ Collaborative Problem	Expected Outcome (The Patient Is Expected to...)	Met/ Not Met	Reason	Date/ Initials
Pain	State that pain is relieved following appropriate interventions			
Potential for postoperative complications (hemorrhage, wound infection, intestinal obstruction, peritonitis, pneumonia/atelectasis)	Have Hgb and Hct WNL, WBC WNL, VS stable, incision clean and dry, clear breath sounds, active bowel sounds			

Aspect of Care	Date ___ Pre-admission/ Pre-op	Date ___ Day 1 (DOS)	Date ___ Day 2 (POD #1)	Date ___ Day 3 (POD #2)	Date ___ Day 4 (POD #3)	Date ___ Day 5–6 (POD #4–5)
Assessment	Systems assessment Pre-op check list Psychosocial assessment	*PACU:* Systems assessment Pain assessment VS q 15 min x 4, q 30 min x 4 until stable Check abdominal dressing with VS checks *Post-op:* Systems assessment Pain assessment	Systems assessment, with focus on breath and bowel sounds Pain assessment VS q 4 h Check abdominal dressing for drainage; assess abdomen for rigidity and distention	Same as Day 2 Check incision after MD removes dressing	VS q 8 h if stable Pain assessment Check abdominal incision for S/S infection and intactness	Same as Day 4 Assess for BM by discharge

		Check abdominal dressing with VS checks Check for voiding				
Teaching	Review clinical pathway/plan of care with patient and family Reinforce pre-op teaching regarding procedure, incision, pain management, and post-op expectations	Teach/demonstrate procedure for DB & C; incentive spirometer Reinforce basic understanding of surgical procedure	Teach additional pain relief measures such as muscle relaxation and visual imagery	Same as Day 2	Begin discharge teaching regarding • Wound care • Pain management • Physical activity • Meds • Complications • When to call MD	Review discharge instructions (verbal and written)
Consults	N/A	Social worker Respiratory therapy	N/A	N/A	N/A	N/A
Lab Tests	Admission labs, including CBC with diff, SMA-6 (6/60), INR(PT)/APTT Type and crossmatch	Hgb and Hct in PM	CBC, lytes	Repeat CBC, lytes if low	N/A	N/A
Other Tests	Colonoscopy, per MD preference Chest x-ray and ECG if >40 years old or history of cardiac disease	N/A	N/A	N/A	N/A	N/A
Meds	One gallon GoLYTELY	PCA with meperidine or morphine	Same as Day 1	D/C PCA; switch to IM or PO opioid, such as Percocet	Same as Day 3	Same as Day 4

Continued

Clinical Pathway for Colon Resection (Without Ostomy) *Continued*

Aspect of Care (Cont'd)	Date ___ Pre-admission/ Pre-op	Date ___ Day 1 (DOS)	Date ___ Day 2 (POD #1)	Date ___ Day 3 (POD #2)	Date ___ Day 4 (POD #3)	Date ___ Day 5–6 (POD #4–5)
Meds (Cont'd)	Neomycin or erythromycin Pre-anesthesia meds	Antibiotic IVPB q 6–8 h x 24 h Antiemetic IM or IV push PRN Tylenol suppository for fever		(Tylox) 2 tabs q 3 h PRN Tylenol 2 tabs PRN for pain/fever Antiemetic PRN		
Treatments/ Interventions	N/A	Thigh-high anti-embolism stockings SCDs or Venodynes to LE I & O q 8 h Catheterize if unable to void 8 h after surgery Frequent mouth care TCDB q 2 h; incentive spirometer q 2 h W/A Teach patient to splint incision Provide emotional support Ankle pumps and ROM to LE q 2 h to prevent thromboembolitic complications	Same as Day 1 Cath PRN Reinforce abdominal dressing PRN	Incision care BID with NS; cover with sterile gauze if incision draining I & O q 8 h VS q 8 h	D/C I & O Incision care VS q 8 h	Same as Day 4

Nutrition	Clear liquids the day before surgery, then NPO	NPO	NPO	Sips H$_2$O → Clear liquids	Clear liquids → full liquids	Progress to DAT
Lines/Tubes/ Monitors	N/A	Continuous IV fluids (Lactated Ringer's → 5% D/$\frac{1}{2}$NS with KCl; MVI if needed) NGT to low suction	Same as Day 1	Clamp NGT Continue with IV fluids	Remove NGT if tolerating liquids D/C IV if taking fluids without nausea	N/A
Mobility/Self-Care	Activity ad lib	Bed rest HOB elevated to at least 30° Assist with ADLs as needed	Up in chair BID Assist with ADLs as needed	Ambulate in room with supervision, if ambulatory Assist with ADLs as needed	Up ad lib; walk into hall	Same as Day 4
Discharge Planning	N/A	Assess for discharge planning to home or other setting Assess personal support systems and financial status	Same as Day 1	Discuss discharge plans with patient and family	Arrange for home health services if needed	Arrange for follow-up appointment as MD specified

Clinical Pathway for Ileostomy/Colostomy

ICD-9 Code **562.10/V44.2/V44.5**   **ELOS 5 days**

Nursing Diagnosis/ Collaborative Problem	Expected Outcome (The Patient Is Expected to...)	Met/ Not Met	Reason	Date/ Initials
Pain	State that pain is relieved following appropriate interventions			
Potential for postoperative complications (hemorrhage, wound infection, intestinal obstruction, peritonitis, pneumonia, atelectasis)	Have Hgb and Hct WNL, WBC WNL, VS stable, incision clean and dry, stoma pink and moist, clear breath sounds, active bowel sounds			
Knowledge deficit regarding ostomy care	Demonstrate the essential care necessary for an ostomy			

Aspect of Care	Date ___ Pre-admission/ Pre-op	Date ___ Day 1 (DOS)	Date ___ Day 2 (POD #1)	Date ___ Day 3 (POD #2)	Date ___ Day 4 (POD #3)	Date ___ Day 5 (POD #4)
Assessment	Systems assessment Pre-op checklist Psychosocial assessment Assess for stoma placement	*PACU:* Systems assessment Pain assessment VS q 15 min x 4, then q 30 min x 4 until stable Check abdominal dressing with VS	Systems assessment with focus on breath and bowel sounds Pain assessment VS q 4 h Check abdominal dressing for drainage; assess abdomen for rigidity and distention	Same as Day 2	VS q 8 h if stable Pain assessment Check abdominal incision for S/S infection and intactness	Same as Day 4 Assess for BM by discharge

Teaching	Review clinical pathway/plan of care with patient and family; Begin teaching about stoma/ostomy care; Reinforce pre-op teaching regarding procedure, incision, stoma, pain management, and post-op expectations	*Post-op:* Systems assessment; Pain assessment; Check abdominal dressing with VS; VS q 1 h x 4, then q 4 h; Check for voiding; Teach/demonstrate procedure for DB & C; incentive spirometer; Reinforce basic understanding of surgical procedure	Check color of stoma; Teach additional pain relief measures, such as muscle relaxation and visual imagery	Same as Day 2	Begin discharge teaching regarding • Wound care • Pain management • Physical activity • Meds • Complications • When to call MD • Ostomy care • Diet therapy	Review discharge instructions (verbal and written)
Consults	Enterostomal therapist	Social worker; Respiratory therapy	N/A	N/A	Dietician	N/A
Lab Tests	Admission labs, including CBC with diff, SMA-6 (6/60), INR(PT)/APTT	Hgb and Hct in PM	CBC, lytes	Repeat CBC, lytes if low	N/A	N/A

Continued

Clinical Pathway for Ileostomy/Colostomy Continued

Aspect of Care (Cont'd)	Date___ Pre-admission/Pre-op	Date___ Day 1 (DOS)	Date___ Day 2 (POD #1)	Date___ Day 3 (POD #2)	Date___ Day 4 (POD #3)	Date___ Day 5 (POD #4)
Other Tests	Colonoscopy, per MD preference Chest x-ray and ECG if >40 years old or history of cardiac disease Abdominal x-ray	N/A	N/A	N/A	N/A	N/A
Meds	One gallon GoLYTELY Neomycin or erythromycin Pre-anesthesia meds	PCA with meperidine or morphine Antibiotic IVPB q 6–8 h x 24 h Antiemetic IM or IV push PRN Tylenol supp for fever	Same as Day 1	D/C PCA; switch to IM or PO opioid, such as Percocet (Tylox) 2 tabs q 3 h PRN Tylenol 2 tabs PRN for pain/fever Antiemetic PRN	Same as Day 3	Same as Day 4
Treatments/ Interventions	N/A	Antiembolism (thigh-high) stockings SCDs or Venodynes to LE I & O q 8 h Catheterize if unable to void within 8 h of surgery Frequent mouth care TCDB q 2 h; incentive spirometer q 2 h W/A (teach patient to splint incision)	Same as Day 1 Cath PRN Reinforce abdominal dressing PRN	Incision care BID with NS; cover with sterile gauze if incision draining Change ostomy pouch and check stoma and peristomal skin I & O q 8 h	D/C I & O Incision care Stoma care	Same as Day 4

		Ankle pumps and ROM to LE q 2 h to prevent thrombolitic complications; Provide emotional support				
Nutrition	Clear liquids the day before surgery, then NPO	NPO	NPO	Sips H$_2$O → clear liquids	Clear liquids → full liquids	Progress to DAT
Lines/Tubes/Monitors	N/A	Continuous IV fluids (Lactated Ringer's → 5% D/½NS with KCl; MVI if needed); NGT to low suction	Same as Day 1	Clamp NGT; Continue with IV fluids	Remove NGT if tolerating liquids; D/C IV if taking fluids without nausea	N/A
Mobility/Self-Care	N/A	Bed rest; HOB elevated to at least 30°; Assist with ADLs as needed; Leg exercises q 2 h	Up in chair BID; Assist with ADLs as needed; Leg exercises q 2 h	Ambulate in room with supervision if ambulatory; Assist with ADLs as needed	Up ad lib; walk into hall	Same as Day 4
Discharge Planning	N/A	Assess for discharge planning to home or other setting; Assess personal support systems and financial status	Discuss discharge plans with patient and family	Same as Day 1	Arrange for home health services if needed	Arrange for follow-up appointment as MD specified

Clinical Pathway for Laennec's Cirrhosis (Without Variceal Bleeding)

ICD-9 Code 571.5   ELOS 3 days

Nursing Diagnosis/ Collaborative Problem	Expected Outcome (The Patient Is Expected to...)	Met/ Not Met	Reason	Date/ Initials
Fluid volume excess (ascites)	Have a decrease in extra-vascular and intra-abdominal fluid as evidenced by decreased abdominal girth and decreased peripheral edema			
Potential for/actual chronic confusion	Be oriented to time, place, and person			
Potential for major complications (esophageal varices, renal failure, advanced encephalopathy)	Not experience bleeding; have renal function tests at or near baseline; have intact neurologic function			

Aspect of Care	Date_____ Day 1	Date_____ Day 2	Date_____ Day 3
Assessment	VS q 4 h if stable / Systems assessment with focus on breath sounds, abdomen, and skin / Assess mental state q 8 h / Observe for bruisability or frank bleeding / Measure abdominal girth QD	Same as Day 1	Same as Day 2
Teaching	Orient to hospital and unit / Review clinical pathway/plan of care with patient and family	Reinforce relationship of alcohol consumption to cirrhosis	Reinforce discharge instructions from Day 2

	Day 1	Day 2	Day 3
	Review diagnosis, including etiology and expected treatment	Review discharge instructions regarding • Drug therapy (diuretics, H$_2$-receptor antagonist) • Avoidance of meds other than prescribed • Diet therapy • Rest • Alcohol abstinence • Fluid restriction	N/A
Consults	Respiratory therapy Alcohol counselor Social worker	N/A	N/A
Lab Tests	CBC, AST, ALT, LDH, alkaline phosphatase, bilirubin, serum proteins, ammonia, prothrombin time, lytes Urine studies for urobilinogen Stool for urobilinogen	N/A	Transaminases, prothrombin time, CBC, ammonia
Other Tests	Chest x-ray ECG Abdominal x-ray/CT of abdomen	N/A	N/A
Meds	Diuretics as needed, such as Lasix IVP or PO Zantac 150 mg BID MVI QD Antacids PRN, such as Riopan or Amphogel Lactulose for ↑ ammonia	Same as Day 1	Same as Day 2

Continued

Clinical Pathway for Laennec's Cirrhosis (Without Variceal Bleeding) Continued

Aspect of Care (Cont'd)	Date ___ Day 1	Date ___ Day 2	Date ___ Day 3
Meds (Cont'd)	Neomycin for ↑ ammonia IV albumin if low serum albumin		
Treatments/Interventions	O₂ PRN for dyspnea Paracentesis if needed for comfort Daily wt I & O q 8 h Fluid restriction to 1500 mL/day Skin care for dryness and jaundice	O₂ PRN Daily wt I & O Fluid restriction Skin care	Same as Day 2
Nutrition	High protein, low → moderate fat, high carbohydrate diet (Low protein diet if ammonia level ↑)	Same as Day 1	Same as Day 2
Lines/Tubes/Monitors	IV at 50 mL/h, then convert to saline loc	Saline loc	D/C saline loc
Mobility/Self-Care	Up in chair BID Keep HOB ↑ to promote breathing comfort Keep feet elevated while patient OOB Assist with ADLs as needed	Walk in room with supervision HOB ↑ Feet ↑ when OOB Assist with ADLs	Same as Day 2
Discharge Planning	Assess home environment and available support systems Determine need for placement in NH or other supervised environment	If discharged to home, make arrangements with home health services to follow patient If discharged to NH or other facility, make transportation and admission arrangements, if not done	Arrange for follow-up appointment with MD as specified

Notes

Clinical Pathway for Cholecystectomy (Open with Common Bile Duct Exploration)

ICD-9 Code **575.0/51.22**   **ELOS 3 days**

Nursing Diagnosis/ Collaborative Problem	Expected Outcome (The Patient Is Expected to...)	Met/ Not Met	Reason	Date/ Initials
Pain	State that chest pain is relieved following appropriate interventions			
Potential for ineffective breathing pattern	Return to baseline respiratory rate and pattern with no adventitious breath sounds			
Potential for postoperative complications (hemorrhage, infection)	Have Hgb and Hct WNL, stable VS, WBC WNL, incision clean and dry, patent and intact T-tube			
Knowledge deficit	Demonstrate care and maintenance of T-tube			

Aspect of Care	Date___ Pre-admission/Pre-op	Date___ Day 1 (DOS)	Date___ Day 2 (POD #1)	Date___ Day 3 (POD #2)
Assessment	Systems assessment Pre-op checklist Psychosocial assessment	*PACU:* Systems assessment Pain assessment VS q 15 min x 4, q 30 min x 4 Check RUQ (abdominal) dressing for drainage; check JP drain	VS QID; check abdominal dressing, JP drain and T-tube Breath sounds and bowel sounds q 8 h	VS q 8 h Assess incision for S/S of infection; assess T-tube insertion site for S/S of infection Assess for BM Breath sounds assessment

	Assess T-tube for patency and drainage (bile) *Post-op:* Pain assessment VS q 1 h x 4, then q 4 h Check dressing and T-tube with VS checks; check JP or other drain Systems assessment Assess for voiding			
Teaching	Review clinical pathway/plan of care with patient and family Pre-op teaching regarding high abdominal incision, need to DB & C, pain management, drains, and general post-op expectations	Orient to hospital and unit Involve family in teaching as appropriate Teach/demonstrate procedure for DB & C (splint incision); incentive spirometer Remind patient to report uncontrolled pain Reinforce basic understanding of surgical procedure	Teach additional pain relief measures such as muscle relaxation and visual imagery Start discharge teaching	Review discharge instructions regarding • Wound care • Pain management • Physical activity • Meds • Dietary restrictions • T-tube care • Complications
Consults	N/A	Respiratory therapy, if indicated, for aggressive pulmonary toilet Social worker	Dietician, if indicated, for weight reduction diet or fat restriction	N/A
Lab Tests	Admission labs INR(PT)/APTT	Hgb and Hct in PM or AM of POD #1	N/A	CBC if Hgb and Hct ↓ WBC count if temp ↑

Continued

Clinical Pathway for Cholecystectomy (Open with Common Bile Exploration) *Continued*

Aspect of Care (Cont'd)	Date ___ Pre-admission/Pre-op	Date ___ Day 1 (DOS)	Date ___ Day 2 (POD #1)	Date ___ Day 3 (POD #2)
Other Tests	Chest x-ray ECG, if >40 years old or history of cardiac disease	Operative cholangiogram	N/A	N/A
Meds	Prophylactic antibiotic at least 1 h before OR Pre-anesthesia meds	PCA or IM meperidine (no morphine) Antiemetic PRN Antibiotic IVPB x 2–3 doses	D/C PCA; continue with IM or PO opioid such as Percocet (Tylox) q 3–4 h PRN	Fleet's enema, laxative, or suppository if no BM by discharge
Treatments/ Interventions	Emotional support; encourage ventilation of feelings about upcoming surgery	I & O q 8 h TCDB with incentive spirometer q 2 h W/A; q 4 h during night Reinforce abdominal dressing PRN Emotional support; encourage ventilation of feelings about surgery	D/C I & O when IV out TCDB Reinforce abdominal dressing PRN Emotional support	MD to change or remove dressing
Nutrition	Low fat diet, then NPO 8 h before OR	NPO except ice chips or sips of H_2O sparingly	Clear → full liquids; progress as tolerated if bowel sounds present	DAT (may need to restrict ↑ fat foods)
Lines/Tubes/Monitors	N/A	Continuous IV fluids JP or other drain (assess drainage, empty and measure q 8 h) T-tube (assess drainage, empty and measure q 8 h; keep drainage bag below level of abdomen at all times)	D/C IV fluids when patient voids and takes adequate fluids JP drainage T-tube to straight drainage	MD may remove JP drain T-tube to straight drainage

			Same as Day 2
Mobility/Self-Care	Activity ad lib	Up in chair with assistance in PM Ankle pumps and ROM to LE q 8 h to prevent thromboembolitic complications; may wear thigh-high antiembolism stockings and/or SCDs	Progressive ambulation May shower (per MD's order)	
Discharge Planning	N/A	Assess home situation for caregiver support and financial status	Reassess home needs and support Arrange for home health services if patient needs assistance with care	Arrange for follow-up appointment as MD specified Arrange for T-tube cholangiogram as outpatient, when MD specified

Clinical Pathway for Peritonitis

ICD-9 Code **567.9**   ELOS **4 days**

Nursing Diagnosis/ Collaborative Problem	Expected Outcome (The Patient Is Expected to...)	Met/ Not Met	Reason	Date/ Initials
Potential for complications (shock, renal failure, sepsis, respiratory failure)	Return to baseline VS; CBC WNL, normal breath sounds; adequate renal function			
Pain	State that pain is relieved after appropriate interventions			
Fluid volume deficit	Be well-hydrated and have normal electrolyte values			

Aspect of Care	Date____ Day 1	Date____ Day 2	Date____ Day 3–4
Assessment	VS q 2–4 h (progress to q 4 h when stabilized) Systems assessment q 8 h Abdominal assessment q 8 h Assess for flatus or BM Assess wound/caths for irrigation, if present, q 8 h Check breath sounds q 8 h	VS q 4 h Systems assessment q 8 h Abdominal assessment q 8 h Assess for flatus or BM Assess wound/caths for irrigation, if present, q 8 h Check breath sounds q 8 h	VS q 8 h Systems assessment q 8 h Abdominal assessment q 8 h Assess for flatus or BM Assess wound/caths for irrigation, if present, q 8 h Check breath sounds q 8 h
Teaching	Orient to hospital and unit Review clinical pathway/plan of care with patient and family Review what peritonitis is and treatment plan	Review diagnosis Review drug information Begin discharge teaching regarding • Drug therapy • Activity restrictions	Review discharge teaching

	Day 1	Day 2	Day 3
		Teach side effects of antibiotics and ask patient to report them if they occur	• S/S to report, such as ↑ temp, ↑ pain, abdominal distention • Diet restrictions, if any
Consults	Infectious diseases Respiratory therapy, if compromise from distention	N/A	N/A
Lab Tests	CBC with diff SMA-6, Cr ABGs Urine for C & S Peritoneal fluid C & S	CBC with diff SMA-6	CBC with diff SMA-6
Other Tests	Abdominal x-ray Chest x-ray and ECG, if >40 years old or history of cardiac disease	N/A	N/A
Meds	IV antibiotics (broad-spectrum followed by specific based on C & S results) Oral analgesic q 3–4 h PRN after definitive diagnosis Intraperitoneal antibiotics Antiemetic PRN for nausea	Same as Day 1	Same as Day 2, then switch to PO antibiotic therapy, if available
Treatments/Interventions	I & O q 8 h If wound for drainage or post-laparotomy, monitor dressing and reinforce as needed Irrigate NGT q 4 h and PRN with NS	Same as Day 1	If wound present, clean with NS BID Irrigate abdominal cath(s) with NS q 8 h, if present I & O

Continued

Clinical Pathway for Peritonitis *Continued*

Aspect of Care (Cont'd)	Date _____ Day 1	Date _____ Day 2	Date _____ Day 3–4
	Irrigate abdominal cath(s) with NS q 8 h, if present Deep breathing/incentive spirometer q 2 h		MD to change dressing, if present Deep breathing/incentive spirometer q 2 h
Nutrition	NPO	Clear liquids (if NGT D/C'd) NPO if NGT continued	Full liquids → DAT
Lines/Tubes/Monitors	NGT to low continuous suction or high intermittent suction (Salem Sump) IV for continuous fluids and antibiotics Abdominal cath(s) (such as Tenchoff) for antibiotic therapy (intraperitoneal)	D/C NGT if ↓ abdominal distention and nausea Continuous IV fluids	Convert IV to saline loc for antibiotic therapy, then D/C saline loc
Mobility/Self-Care	Bed rest with BRP (if not too weak) HOB in semi-Fowler's position at all times	Up in chair with assistance BID Keep in semi-Fowler's position	Begin ambulation in room with supervision
Discharge Planning	Assess home environment and support systems	If home health services needed, arrange for services from nursing or homemaker assistance	Continue as Day 2

Notes

Unit

VII

Problems Affecting Women's Health/ Reproductive Health Problems

▼ ▼ ▼

Clinical Pathway for Total Abdominal Hysterectomy

ICD-9 Code 218.9/68.4   ELOS 3 days

Nursing Diagnosis/ Collaborative Problem	Expected Outcome (The Patient Is Expected to...)	Met/ Not Met	Reason	Date/ Initials
Pain	State that pain is relieved following appropriate interventions			
Potential for postoperative complications (hemorrhage, infection)	Have Hgb and Hct WNL, stable VS, and WBC WNL; incision clean and dry			
Potential for ineffective coping/body image disturbance	Participate in self-care, ventilate feelings about effects of surgery, and identify support systems			

Aspect of Care	Date____ Pre-admission/Pre-op	Date____ Day 1 (DOS)	Date____ Day 2 (POD #1)	Date____ Day 3 (POD #2)
Assessment	Systems assessment Pre-op checklist Psychosocial assessment	*PACU:* Systems assessment Pain assessment VS q 15 min x 4, q 30 min x 4 Check abdominal dressing for drainage Assess vaginal discharge with VS checks *Post-op:* Pain assessment	VS QID Monitor abdominal dressing Breath sounds and bowel sounds q 8 h Check for spontaneous voiding after Foley removal	VS q 8 h Assess incision for S/S of infection Assess for BM

(Assessment)		VS q 1 h x 4, then q 4 h Check abdominal dressing and vaginal discharge with VS checks Systems assessment		
Teaching	Pre-op teaching regarding surgical procedure, incision, pain management, and post-op expectations Review plan of care/clinical pathway with patient and family	Orient to hospital and unit Teach/demonstrate procedure for DB & C and incentive spirometer Remind patient to report excessive bleeding or severe pain Reinforce basic understanding of surgical procedure	Teach additional pain relief measures, such as muscle relaxation and visual imagery Teach perineal care procedure	Review discharge instructions regarding • Wound care • Pain management • Physical activity • Sexual activity • Complications • Physical changes • Meds
Consults	N/A	Social worker	N/A	N/A
Lab Tests	Admission labs INR(PT)/APTT	Hgb and Hct in PM or next AM	N/A	N/A
Other Tests	Chest x-ray and ECG if >40 years old or history of cardiac disease	N/A	N/A	N/A
Meds	Prophylactic antibiotic at least 1 h before OR Pre-anesthesia meds	PCA with meperidine or morphine until POD #1 AM Antiemetic PRN Toradol IM PRN for breakthrough pain Antibiotic IVPB q 6–8 h x 3–4 doses	D/C PCA; switch to Percocet (Tylox) PO or other opioid q 3–4 h PRN	Percocet or other opoid q 3–4 h PRN Fleet's enema or suppository if no BM before discharge

Continued

Clinical Pathway for Total Abdominal Hysterectomy *Continued*

Aspect of Care (Cont'd)	Date _____ Pre-admission/Pre-op	Date _____ Day 1 (DOS)	Date _____ Day 2 (POD #1)	Date _____ Day 3 (POD #2)
Treatments/ Interventions	N/A	I & O x 24 h Perineal care q 4 h W/A DB & C q 2 h with incentive spirometer Reinforce abdominal dressing PRN Emotional support; encourage ventilation of feelings about surgery and body image effects	Perineal care q 8 h (patient may do own) DB & C q 2 h with incentive spirometer Reinforce abdominal dressing PRN	Same as Day 2 (POD #1) MD to change or remove dressing
Nutrition	NPO after 12 midnight	NPO except ice chips or sips of H_2O sparingly	Clear → full liquids; progress as tolerated if bowel sounds present	DAT
Lines/Tubes/Monitors	N/A	Continuous IV fluids Foley cath Monitor Foley output and measure q 8 h	D/C Foley if urine clear and output adequate D/C IV fluids when patient voids and takes adequate PO fluids without nausea	N/A
Mobility/Self-Care	Activity ad lib	Dangle at bedside; up in chair with assistance in PM if early AM surgery Thigh-high antiembolism stockings; ankle pumps and LE ROM q 2 h	Progressive ambulation May shower (per MD's order) Thigh-high antiembolism stockings	Same as Day 2
Discharge Planning	N/A	Assess home situation for support systems and financial status	Reassess home needs and support	Arrange for follow-up appointment as MD specified Home health referral if patient is unable to provide self-care

Notes

Clinical Pathway for Total Vaginal Hysterectomy

ICD-9 Code 218.9/68.5   **ELOS 3 days**

Nursing Diagnosis/Collaborative Problem	Expected Outcome (The Patient Is Expected to...)	Met/Not Met	Reason	Date/Initials
Pain	State that pain is relieved following appropriate interventions			
High risk for postoperative complications (hemorrhage, infection)	Have Hgb and Hct WNL, stable VS, WBC WNL, and clear yellow urine			
High risk for infective individual coping	Participate in self-care, express feelings about effects of surgery, and identify support systems			

Aspect of Care	Date_____ Pre-admission/Pre-op	Date_____ Day 1 (DOS)	Date_____ Day 2 (POD #1)	Date_____ Day 3 (POD #2)
Assessment	Systems assessment Pre-op checklist Psychosocial assessment	*PACU:* Systems assessment Pain assessment VS q 15 min x 4, then q 30 min x 4 Vaginal bleeding checks with VS; pad count *Post-op:* Pain assessment VS q 1 h x 4, then q 4 h	VS QID; assess vaginal bleeding with VS; pad count Breath sounds and bowel sounds q 8 h Pain assessment	VS q 8 h; assess vaginal bleeding Breath sounds and bowel sounds q 8 h Assess for BM

Vaginal bleeding checks with VS; pad count
Systems assessment

Teaching	Pre-op teaching regarding surgery, pain management, and post-op expectations; Review plan of care/clinical pathway with patient and family	Orient to hospital and unit; Teach/demonstrate procedure for DB & C, incentive spirometer; Remind patient to expect heavy vaginal bleeding initially and to report passing large clots or having severe pain; Reinforce basic understanding of surgical procedure	Teach additional pain relief measures such as muscle relaxation and visual imagery; Teach measures to prevent thromboembolitic complications, such as ankle pumps and ROM to LE; Teach perineal care procedure	Review discharge instructions regarding • Pain management • Foley or suprapubic cath care (possible clamping schedule) • Physical activity • Sexual activity • Physical changes • Meds
Consults	Social worker	N/A	N/A	N/A
Lab Tests	Admission labs; INR(PT)/APTT	Hgb and Hct	N/A	N/A
Other Tests	Chest x-ray and ECG if >40 years old or history of cardiac disease	N/A	N/A	N/A
Meds	Prophylactic antibiotic at least 1 h before OR; Pre-anesthesia meds	PCA or IM meperidine or morphine until POD #1; Antiemetic PRN	D/C PCA or IMs; switch to Percocet (Tylox) or other PO opioid q 3–4 h PRN; Stool softener at bedtime	Percocet or other oral opioid 3–4 hr PRN; Fleet's enema or suppository if no BM by discharge
Treatments/ Interventions	Emotional support; encourage ventilation of feelings about surgery, body image, loss	I & O x 24 h; Perineal care q 4 h and after toileting	Perineal care (patient may do own)	Perineal care; Sitz baths

Continued

Clinical Pathway for Total Vaginal Hysterectomy Continued

Aspect of Care (Cont'd)	Date_____ Pre-admission/Pre-op	Date_____ Day 1 (DOS)	Date_____ Day 2 (POD #1)	Date_____ Day 3 (POD #2)
Treatments/ Interventions (Cont'd)		DB & C q 2 h with incentive spirometer Emotional support	Remove vaginal packing Sitz baths PRN	
Nutrition	NPO 8 hrs before OR	NPO except ice chips or sips of H_2O sparingly	Clear → full liquids; progress as tolerated if BS present	DAT
Lines/Tubes/Monitors	N/A	Foley or suprapubic urinary cath Continuous IV fluids Irrigate PRN with NS Monitor output q 8 h	D/C IV fluids when tolerating fluids and no nausea Continue with Foley/suprapubic cath; measure and note output q 8 h	Foley/suprapubic cath
Mobility/Self-Care	Activity ad lib	Dangle at bedside; up in chair with assistance in PM if early AM surgery Thigh-high antiembolism stockings; ankle pumps and LE ROM q 2 h	Progressive ambulation May shower (per MD's order) Thigh-high antiembolism stockings	Same as Day 2
Discharge Planning	N/A	Assess home situation for support systems and financial status	Reassess home needs and support	Arrange for follow-up appointment as MD specified Home health referral if patient is discharged with Foley cath and unable to provide self-care

Notes

Clinical Pathway for Mastectomy (Modified Radical)

ICD-9 Code 174.9/85.43   ELOS 3 days

Nursing Diagnosis/ Collaborative Problem	Expected Outcome (The Patient Is Expected to...)	Met/ Not Met	Reason	Date/ Initials
Pain	State that pain is relieved following appropriate interventions			
High risk for postoperative complications (edema, infection, hemorrhage, hematoma)	Have Hgb and Hct WNL, stable VS, WBC WNL, incision clean and dry, no unusual swelling			
Ineffective individual coping	Look at incision before discharge; identify individual and family coping strategies that have been successful in the past			
Impaired physical mobility (affected arm and shoulder)	Perform prescribed exercises to improve mobility of affected arm and shoulder			

Aspect of Care	Date ___ Pre-admission/Pre-op	Date ___ Day 1 (DOS)	Date ___ Day 2 (POD #1)	Date ___ Day 3 (POD #2)
Assessment	Systems assessment Pre-op checklist Psychosocial assessment	*PACU:* Systems assessment Pain assessment VS q 15 min x 4, then q 30 min x 4 Assess surgical dressing and drain (JP/Hemovac)	VS q 8 h Breath sounds q 8 h Assess dressing and drain with VS	VS BID Monitor incision for S/S of infection, hematoma, or swelling

		Post-op: Pain assessment VS q 1 h x 4, then q 4 h Assess dressing and drain with VS checks Systems assessments		
Teaching	Pre-op teaching regarding incision drain, pain, and post-op expectations Review plan of care/clinical pathway with patient and family	Orient to hospital and unit Teach patient • To avoid having procedures such as BP and venipuncture in affected arm (post sign over bed) • About Reach to Recovery services • How to do flexion and extension of fingers and wrist of affected arm	Encourage patient to use upright posture and have arms by side while walking and standing Demonstrate/teach early mastectomy exercises for affected arm, such as ROM for hand, wrist, and elbow, and touching hand to shoulder Teach additional pain relief measures, such as muscle relaxation and visual imagery	Reinforce exercises and remind patient to start abduction, ROM to shoulder, and squeezing a ball after 1 wk Teach importance of avoiding injury to affected arm, including shaving of underarm or deodorant topical creams or ointments Teach/review discharge instructions regarding • Wound care • Pain management (including nondrug measures) • Physical activity • S/S of infection • BSE and mammography (opposite breast) and JP drain management (if not removed before discharge)
Consults	N/A	Social worker	N/A	N/A
Lab Tests	Admission labs, including CBC, SMA-6, INR(PT)/APTT	N/A	N/A	N/A

Continued

Clinical Pathway for Mastectomy (Modified Radical) *Continued*

Aspect of Care (Cont'd)	Date_____ Pre-admission/Pre-op	Date_____ Day 1 (DOS)	Date_____ Day 2 (POD #1)	Date_____ Day 2 (POD #2)
Other Tests	ECG and chest x-ray for >40 years old or history of cardiac disease	N/A	N/A	N/A
Meds	Prophylactic antibiotic at least 1 h before OR Pre-anesthesia meds	IM meperidine or morphine, or PO Percocet (Tylox) q 3–4 h PRN	Continue with PO pain med PRN	Same as Day 2
Treatments/ Interventions	Emotional support OR prep	I & O until taking fluids and voided DB & C Incentive spirometer q 2 h HOB at least 30° Position on back or unaffected side with affected operative side arm elevated slightly on pillow while in bed Reinforce dressing if needed	Continue measuring drainage from JP q 8 h	Continue to elevate affected arm on pillow when not exercising MD to remove or change dressing
Nutrition	NPO after 12 midnight	NPO until fully awake, then clear liquids and advance as tolerated	DAT	Same as Day 2
Lines/Tubes/Monitors	N/A	D/C IV fluids when voided and taking adequate liquids Monitor drainage from JP drain	N/A	MD to remove drain if <30 mL drainage in 24 h

Mobility/Self-Care	Activity ad lib	Up in chair and to BR with assistance	Progressive ambulation Encourage gentle use of affected arm for ADLs	Same as Day 2
Discharge Planning	N/A	Assess coping ability Contact Reach for Recovery with patient's permission Assess home situation, including support systems	Reassess home needs and support Provide American Cancer Society materials/pamphlets	Arrange for follow-up appointment as MD specified Arrange for radiation therapy or chemotherapy, if indicated Encourage new support systems, such as community support groups Provide information about availability of temporary or permanent prosthesis Encourage patient to discuss options for breast reconstruction with MD

Unit

VIII

Other Health Problems

Clinical Pathway for Cellulitis

ICD-9 Code **682.6**   **ELOS 4 days**

Nursing Diagnosis/Collaborative Problem	Expected Outcome (The Patient Is Expected to...)	Met/Not Met	Reason	Date/Initials
Impaired skin integrity	Experience initial healing of skin and underlying tissues			
Pain	State that pain is relieved after appropriate interventions			
Knowledge deficit	Describe skin care needed to prevent further episodes of cellulitis, if cognitively intact			
Impaired physical mobility	Ambulate in hall with supervision (may require walker), if ambulatory			

Aspect of Care	Date____ Day 1	Date____ Day 2	Date____ Day 3	Date____ Day 4
Assessment	Skin/wound assessment q 8 h VS q 4 h Pain assessment with VS Risk factor assessment (diabetes, PVD, age) Fall risk assessment Family support and resources	Skin/wound assessment q 8 h VS q 4 h Pain assessment with VS	Same as Day 2	Same as Day 3

Teaching	Review relationship of risk factors to cellulitis Teach importance of proper nutrition for healing Review purpose and side effects of meds Begin/reinforce diabetic teaching, if diabetic Review plan of care/clinical pathway with patient and family	Continue with diabetic teaching, if indicated	Same as Day 2	Review discharge instructions regarding • Wound/skin care • Meds • Physical activity • Handwashing and other infection control measures
Consults	Dietician, if needed for diabetic PT, if needed, for ambulation with walker Social worker Infectious disease services, if needed or if available	N/A	N/A	N/A
Lab Tests	CBC with diff, BUN, Cr, glucose, lytes (SMA-6 or 6/60) Wound C & S (for open wound)	Fasting blood sugar, if diabetic	Same as Day 2 Repeat WBC if ↑	Same as Day 3
Other Tests	ECG, chest x-ray, if >40 years old or history of heart disease X-ray of affected area if osteomyelitis suspected	N/A	N/A	N/A

Continued

Clinical Pathway for Cellulitis *Continued*

Aspect of Care (Cont'd)	Date_____ Day 1	Date_____ Day 2	Date_____ Day 3	Date_____ Day 4
Meds	Antibiotics IVPB (broad-spectrum initially until C & S results) Percocet (Tylox) or other PO analgesic q 3–4 h PRN Tylenol PRN for ↑ temp Oral hypoglycemic or sliding scale insulin, if diabetic MVI with iron QD (PO or IV)	Same as Day 1	Same as Day 2	Switch to PO antibiotic Continue with other meds as needed
Treatments/ Interventions	I & O Calorie count for ↓ nutritional status W→D NS dressing change (may be with irrigation) q 8 h, or as MD specified Affected extremity elevated on pillow Wound precautions, for open wound Emotional support; encourage ventilation about diagnosis and coping strategies Fall precautions, if at risk for fall	Same as Day 1	D/C I & O Same as Day 2	Dressing changes q 8 h Extremity evaluation

Nutrition	High protein, high iron diet for healing Diabetic diet, if indicated	Same as Day 1 May need supplemental enteral nutrition, such as Ensure or Glucerna	Same as Day 2	Same as Day 3
Lines/Tubes/Monitors	Continuous IV fluids	Convert to saline loc if PO fluid intake adequate and temp ↓	Saline loc	D/C saline loc
Mobility/Self-Care	Bed rest with BRP or BSC (may need assistance and/or walker) Assist with ADLs as needed	Up in chair BID with affected extremity elevated Assist with ADLs as needed	Ambulate in room with walker (if ambulatory)	Same as Day 3
Discharge Planning	Social worker for possible NH placement or home health	Reassess family support and resources Refer to home health services or NH as needed	Arrange for dressing supplies, equipment to be used at home (for home discharge)	Arrange for follow-up appointment as MD specified

Clinical Pathway for Urosepsis/Dehydration

ICD-9 Code **599.0**   ELOS **4 days**

Nursing Diagnosis/ Collaborative Problem	Expected Outcome (The Patient Is Expected to...)	Met/ Not Met	Reason	Date/ Initials
Fluid volume deficit	Have fluid and electrolyte values WNL			
Hyperthermia	Have temp return to baseline			
Potential for impaired skin integrity	Have intact skin/no new lesions			

Aspect of Care	Date_____ Day 1	Date_____ Day 2	Date_____ Day 3	Date_____ Day 4
Assessment	VS q 4 h (if temp ↑, VS at least q 2 h) Urinary assessment, including frequency and characteristics of urine Skin/wound assessment q 8 h Family support and resources Fall risk assessment Risk factor assessment such as age, mental status, nutritional status Teaching/learning ability	VS q 4 h Skin/wound assessment q 8 h	Same as Day 2	Same as Day 3

Teaching	Orient to hospital and unit Review relationship of sepsis and dehydration Teach process and source of sepsis Teach importance of proper nutrition for healing Review purpose and side effects of meds Review plan of care/clinical pathway with patient and family	Reinforce teaching from Day 1	Same as Day 2	Review discharge instructions regarding: • Fluid intake • Nutrition • Sepsis prevention • Skin/wound care, as needed
Consults	Dietitian, if indicated Social worker, if placement needed Infectious disease service, if needed or if available	N/A	N/A	N/A
Lab Tests	CBC with diff, BUN, Cr, glucose, lytes, SMA-6 or 6/60 Blood culture U/A, urine for C & S	CBC, SMA-6 Repeat blood culture if temp >101°F (37°C)	Repeat WBC, if ↑ Repeat SMA-6, if lytes not WNL	N/A
Other Tests	Chest x-ray ECG	N/A	N/A	N/A
Meds	Antibiotics IVPB (broad-spectrum initially until C & S results) Urinary antiseptic	Same as Day 1	Same as Day 2	Switch to PO antibiotic Continue with pain meds, if needed PRN

Continued

Clinical Pathway for Urosepsis/Dehydration *Continued*

Aspect of Care (Cont'd)	Date ____ Day 1	Date ____ Day 2	Date ____ Day 3	Date ____ Day 4
Meds (Cont'd)	Percocet (Tylox) or other PO analgesic q 3–4 PRN Tylenol PRN for ↑ temp			
Treatments/ Interventions	I & O Mouth and skin care q 8 h Calorie count for ↓ nutritional status Daily wt Turn q 2 h; skin assessment when turning	Same as Day 1	Same as Day 2	Same as Day 3 D/C I & O and calorie count
Nutrition	High protein, high iron, high calorie diet as tolerated Increase PO fluids	Same as Day 1 May need supplemental enteral nutrition, such as Ensure	DAT	DAT
Lines/Tubes/Monitors	Continuous IV fluids for rehydration and electrolyte replacement as needed Foley cath (for urinary retention only)	Same as Day 1	Convert to saline loc if PO fluid intake adequate and temp ↓	D/C saline loc
Mobility/Self-Care	Bed rest Assist with ADLs as needed Fall precautions if at risk for falls	Bed rest with BRP or BSC (may need assistance and/or walker) Up in chair BID Assist with ADLs as needed	May ambulate in room with walker, if able	Same as Day 3

Discharge Planning			
Social worker to assess for placement or referral services	Assess family support and resources Refer to home health services, if indicated Continue to evaluate for NH placement or return to home	Same as Day 2	Arrange for follow-up appointment as MD specified

Clinical Pathway for Stage 1 Pressure Ulcer*

ICD-9 Code 707   ELOS Length of stay often depends on underlying cause and other diagnoses

Nursing Diagnosis/ Collaborative Problem	Expected Outcome (The Patient Is Expected to...)	Met/ Not Met	Reason	Date/ Initials
Alteration in tissue integrity	Have intact skin with no redness			

Aspect of Care	Date ___ Day 1	Date ___ Day 2	Date ___ Day 3	Date ___ Day 4	Date ___ Day 5	Date ___ Day 6
Assessment	Systems assessment q shift; Assess skin integrity especially over bony prominences for reddened areas that do not fade or blanch; Assess need for air mattress, heel and elbow protectors, gel float pads, sheepskin, etc.; VS q 8 h; Psychosocial assessment	Same as Day 1	Same as Day 2	Same as Day 3	Same as Day 4	Same as Day 5
Teaching	Orient to hospital and unit; Provide information concerning pressure ulcers	Continue to provide patient and family information regarding prevention and treatment	Teach patient and family dressing changes, skin care, mobility, diet	Continue as Day 3	Continue as Day 4	Continue as Day 5

*Adapted with permission from Harbor Hospital Center, Baltimore, Maryland. Developed by the Interdisciplinary Wound Care Team.

	Day 1	Day 2	Day 3	Day 4	Day 5	Day 6
	Involve family in care of patient as appropriate Review plan of care/clinical pathway with patient and family					
Consults	Dietician Enterostomal therapist Physical therapist	N/A	N/A	N/A	N/A	N/A
Lab Tests	SMA-20 CBC	N/A	N/A	Protein, albumin	N/A	N/A
Other Tests	N/A	N/A	N/A	N/A	N/A	N/A
Meds	Multivitamin QD	Same as Day 1	Same as Day 2	Same as Day 3	Same as Day 4	Same as Day 5
Treatments/ Interventions	Apply extra thin hydrocolloid to pressure ulcer sites; change q 5 days or as needed for removal or leakage Daily wt I & O *Dry skin:* For bath, use mild soap or very little soap	Evaluate dressing integrity; change if needed Same as Day 1	Same as Day 2	Remeasure and evaluate the pressure ulcer Dressing change PRN	Dressing change PRN	Same as Day 5

Clinical Pathway for Stage 1 Pressure Ulcer *Continued*

Aspect of Care (Cont'd)	Date ___ Day 1	Date ___ Day 2	Date ___ Day 3	Date ___ Day 4	Date ___ Day 5	Date ___ Day 6
Treatments/ Interventions (Cont'd)	*Very dry skin:* Bath oil; apply petroleum jelly lightly to wet skin *Incontinence:* Keep skin clean and dry; use Uniwash, Unisalve and/or cornstarch with each incontinent episode *Fecal incontinence:* Apply fecal pouch; evaluate need for antidiarrheals or disimpaction; use reusable underpads *Urinary incontinence:* If appropriate for males, use male external cath; change incontinent briefs when wet; do not position patient on Foley cath tubing; straight cath q 4 h using sterile technique					

Nutrition	High protein, high calorie unless contraindicted Calorie count Assess need for dietary supplement	High protein, high calorie diet unless contraindicted	Same as Day 2	Same as Day 3	Same as Day 4	Same as Day 5
Lines/Tubes/ Monitors	N/A	N/A	N/A	N/A	N/A	N/A
Mobility/Self- Care	*Immobile / bed rest:* TCDB q 2 h; move by lifting not pulling or dragging ROM q 4 h W/A Avoid positioning on bony prominences/ areas Position the patient on an angle when sidelying Use pillows under lower legs to elevate heels in supine lying and between knees and ankles when in sidelying position Use pillows or foot drop splints to position ankles to prevent contracture	Evaluate mobility level and treat as indicated Same as Day 1	Same as Day 2	Same as Day 3	Same as Day 4	Same as Day 5

Continued

Clinical Pathway for Stage 1 Pressure Ulcer Continued

Aspect of Care (Cont'd)	Date ___ Day 1	Date ___ Day 2	Date ___ Day 3	Date ___ Day 4	Date ___ Day 5	Date ___ Day 6
Mobility/Self-Care (Cont'd)	*Up in chair with assistance:*					
	TCDB q 2 h					
	Encourage wt shifting q 2 h; if patient unable to shift wt, use pillows under ischial tuberosities					
	Use a draw sheet or bath blanket to cover chair					
	If patient in a recliner, change its position q 1 h; use pillows under lower legs when in reclined position					
	Patients with decreased mental status should not sit longer than 4 h					
	Ambulatory requiring assistance:					
	Assist patient with ambulation TID					
	Reposition in bed or chair as needed					
	Ambulatory—independent:					
	Encourage ambulation TID					

Discharge Planning					
Evaluate support systems Evaluate need for preventative equipment and supplies *Discharge home:* Notify home health *Discharge NH:* Notify nursing home of pressure ulcer and treatment measures used on transfer form and in oral report	Continue as Day 1	Continue as Day 2	Evaluate progress of discharge planning and any unmet needs	Continue to resolve any problems identified on Day 4 Ensure that all needed supplies at home have been received	Same as Day 5

Clinical Pathway for Stage 2 Pressure Ulcer*

ICD-9 Code 707   ELOS Length of stay is dependent upon medical condition; patient may be discharged to home or LTC facility for further treatment of the pressure ulcer

Nursing Diagnosis/ Collaborative Problem	Expected Outcome (The Patient Is Expected to...)	Met/ Not Met	Reason	Date/ Initials
Alteration in tissue integrity	Perform wound care and understand how to prevent further occurrence of skin breakdown *or* If the patient is unable to, the family provides the needed care			
Pain	Be free of discomfort or state that pain is controlled with analgesics			

Aspect of Care	Date ___ Day 1	Date ___ Day 2	Date ___ Day 3	Date ___ Day 4	Date ___ Day 5	Date ___ Day 6
Assessment	Systems assessment q shift Assess skin integrity for loss of the first layer of skin (i.e., scratch or blister) • Location • Stage • Size (include areas of redness around the actual ulcer)	Same as Day 1	Same as Day 2	Same as Day 3	Same as Day 4	Same as Day 5

*Adapted with permission from Harbor Hospital Center, Baltimore, Maryland. Developed by the Interdisciplinary Wound Care Team.

	Day	Day 3	Day 4	Day 5
• Color of wound bed • Exudate Assess need for air mattress, heel and elbow protectors, etc. VS q 8 h Psychosocial assessment Assess for contributing factors • Immobility, inactivity • Incontinence • Malnutrition or dehydration • Frailty • Under normal wt or overwt • Diabetes • Anemia • Anascara • Immuno-suppression • Systemic disease				
Teaching Orient to hospital and unit Provide information concerning pressure ulcers Involve family in care of patient as appropriate	Continue to provide patient and family information regarding prevention and treatment	Teach patient and family dressing changes, skin care, mobility, diet	Continue as Day 3	Continue as Day 4
				Continue as Day 5

Continued

Clinical Pathway for Stage 2 Pressure Ulcer *Continued*

Aspect of Care (Cont'd)	Date ___ Day 1	Date ___ Day 2	Date ___ Day 3	Date ___ Day 4	Date ___ Day 5	Date ___ Day 6
Teaching (Cont'd)	Review plan of care/clinical pathway with patient and family					
Consults	Dietician Enterostomal therapist Physical therapist	N/A	N/A	N/A	N/A	N/A
Lab Tests	SMA-6(60) CBC with diff	N/A	N/A	Protein, albumin	N/A	N/A
Other Tests	N/A	N/A	N/A	N/A	N/A	N/A
Meds	Multivitamin QD	Same as Day 1	Same as Day 2	Same as Day 3	Same as Day 4	Same as Day 5
Treatments/ Interventions	Clean wound with NS and dry skin around ulcer gently Suggestions for dressing changes are placed in the order in which they should be tried (all dressing should extend at least $1\frac{1}{4}$ inch beyond the margin of the reddened area) • Extra thin hydrocolloid dressing; change dressing q 3 days	Evaluate dressing integrity; change if needed Same as Day 1	Same as Day 2	Remeasure and evaluate pressure ulcer Dressing change PRN	Dressing change PRN	Same as Day 5

Continued

- Vaseline gauze, xeroform gauze, or bacitracin and gauze; change QD to BID
- Neosporin and gauze
- Gentamicin and gauze
- Silvadene 1% and gauze
- Neomycin and gauze
- Bactroban and gauze

Daily wt

I & O

Dry skin:

For bath, use mild soap or very little soap

Very dry skin:

Bath oil; apply petroleum jelly lightly to wet skin

Incontinence:

Keep skin clean and dry; use Uniwash, Unisalve (or other similar product) and/or cornstarch with each incontinent episode

Clinical Pathway for Stage 2 Pressure Ulcer *Continued*

Aspect of Care (Cont'd)	Date ___ Day 1	Date ___ Day 2	Date ___ Day 3	Date ___ Day 4	Date ___ Day 5	Date ___ Day 6
Treatments/ Interventions (Cont'd)	*Fecal incontinence:* Apply fecal pouch; evaluate need for antidiarrheals or disimpaction; use reusable underpads *Urinary incontinence:* If appropriate for males, use male external cath; change incontinent briefs when wet; do not position patient on Foley cath tubing					
Nutrition	High protein unless contraindicted Calorie count x 3 days Assess need for dietary supplement	High protein diet unless contraindicated	Same as Day 2	Same as Day 3	Same as Day 4	Same as Day 5
Lines/Tubes/ Monitors	N/A	N/A	N/A	N/A	N/A	N/A
Mobility/Self-Care	*Immobile / bed rest:* TCDB q 2 h ROM q 2 h W/A Avoid positioning on bony prominences/ areas	Evaluate mobility level and treat as indicated	Same as Day 2	Same as Day 3	Same as Day 4	Same as Day 5

Continued

Position the patient on an angle when sidelying

Use pillows under lower legs to elevate heels in supine lying and between knees and ankles when in sidelying position

Use pillows or foot drop splints to position ankles to prevent contracture

Up in chair with assistance:

TCDB q 2 h

Encourage wt shifting q 2 h; if patient unable to shift wt, use pillows under ischial tuberosities

Use a draw sheet or bath blanket to cover chair

If patient in a recliner, change its position q 1 h; use pillows under lower legs when in reclined position

Patients with decreased mental status should not sit longer than 4 h

Clinical Pathway for Stage 2 Pressure Ulcer *Continued*

Aspect of Care (Cont'd)	Date ___ Day 1	Date ___ Day 2	Date ___ Day 3	Date ___ Day 4	Date ___ Day 5	Date ___ Day 6
Mobility/Self-Care (Cont'd)	*Ambulatory requiring assistance:* Assist patient with ambulation TID Reposition in bed or chair as needed *Ambulatory—independent:* Encourage ambulation QID					
Discharge Planning	Evaluate support systems Evaluate need for preventative equipment and supplies *Discharge home:* Notify home health *Discharge NH:* Refer to case manager for NH return/referral; notify NH of pressure ulcer and treatment measures used on transfer form and in oral report	Continue as Day 1	Continue as Day 2	Evaluate progress of discharge planning and any unmet needs	Continue to resolve any problems identified on Day 4 Ensure that needed supplies are in the home	Same as Day 5

Notes

Clinical Pathway for Stage 3 Pressure Ulcer*

ICD-9 Code **707.0**   ELOS Length of stay is dependent upon medical condition; patient may be discharged to home or LTC facility for further treatment of the pressure ulcer

Nursing Diagnosis/ Collaborative Problem	Expected Outcome (The Patient Is Expected to...)	Met/ Not Met	Reason	Date/ Initials
Alteration in tissue integrity	Performs wound care and understands how to prevent deterioration and further occurrence of pressure ulcers *or* If the patient is unable to, the family provides the needed care			
Pain	Be free of pain or state that pain is controlled with analgesics			

Aspect of Care	Date____ Day 1	Date____ Day 2	Date____ Day 3	Date____ Day 4	Date____ Day 5	Date____ Day 6
Assessment	Systems assessment q shift Assess skin integrity for ulcer that is deeper than loss of first layer of skin into subcutaneous tissue but not to muscle or bone • Location • Stage	Same as Day 1	Same as Day 2 Measure size of pressure ulcer	Same as Day 3 VS q 8 h	Same as Day 4	Same as Day 5

*Adapted with permission from Harbor Hospital Center, Baltimore, Maryland. Developed by the Interdisciplinary Wound Care Team.

• Size (include areas of redness around the actual ulcer) • Color of wound bed • Exudate Pressure ulcer assessment sheet x 2/week VS q 4 h Psychosocial assessment Assess for contributing factors • Immobility, inactivity • Incontinence • Malnutrition or dehydration • Frailty • Under normal wt or overwt • Diabetes • Anemia • Anascara • Immunosuppression • Systemic disease			Continue as Day 3	Continue as Day 4	Continue as Day 5
Teaching Orient to hospital and unit Provide information concerning pressure ulcers	Continue to provide patient and family information regarding ulcer formation, prevention, and treatment	Teach patient and family dressing changes, skin care, mobility, diet	Continue as Day 3	Continue as Day 4	Continue as Day 5

Continued

Clinical Pathway for Stage 3 Pressure Ulcer Continued

Aspect of Care (Cont'd)	Date ___ Day 1	Date ___ Day 2	Date ___ Day 3	Date ___ Day 4	Date ___ Day 5	Date ___ Day 6
Teaching (Cont'd)	Involve family in care of patient as appropriate Review plan of care/clinical pathway with patient and family					
Consults	Dietician Enterostomal therapist Physical therapist Surgeon	N/A	N/A	N/A	N/A	N/A
Lab Tests	SMA-6(60) CBC Blood culture and gram stain Wound culture and gram stain	N/A	N/A	Blood culture Pressure ulcer culture	CBC, SMA-6(60)	N/A
Other Tests	ECG U/A, C & S Chest x-ray	N/A	N/A	N/A	N/A	N/A
Meds	Multivitamin QD IV/PO antibiotics for wound infection with cellulitis	Same as Day 1	Same as Day 2	Same as Day 3	Same as Day 4	Change to PO antibiotics, if applicable

Treatments/Interventions					
Evaluate need for specialty bed using decision tree Clean wound with NS and dry skin around ulcer gently Dressing changes are placed in the order in which they should be tried • Hydrocolloid gel with or without paste; change QD to BID • Hydroactive gel covered with gauze; if wound has necrotic tissue, change q 2 days; if wound is granulating, gel may remain up to 7 days; gel may be used with a wafer • Silvadene 1% and gauze BID • Chlorapactin and gauze packing, change BID to TID • Algiderm wound packing for draining wounds; cover with gauze and tape and change q 1–5 days; packing may be used under a wafer	Dressing changes as needed	Same as Day 2	Remeasure and evaluate pressure ulcer Dressing change PRN	Dressing change PRN	Same as Day 5

Continued

Clinical Pathway for Stage 3 Pressure Ulcer Continued

Aspect of Care (Cont'd)	Date ___ Day 1	Date ___ Day 2	Date ___ Day 3	Date ___ Day 4	Date ___ Day 5	Date ___ Day 6
Treatments/ Interventions (Cont'd)	Daily wt I & O *Dry skin:* For bath, use mild soap or very little soap *Very dry skin:* Bath oil; apply petroleum jelly lightly to wet skin *Incontinence:* Keep skin clean and dry; use Uniwash, Unisalve (or other similar product) and/or cornstarch with each incontinent episode *Fecal incontinence:* Apply fecal pouch; evaluate need for antidiarrheals or disimpaction; use reusable underpads *Urinary incontinence:* If appropriate for males, use male external cath; change incontinent briefs when wet; do not position patient on Foley cath tubing					

	Day 1	Day 2	Day 3	Day 4	Day 5	Day 6
Nutrition	High protein, high calorie unless contraindicted Encourage fluids Calorie count Assess need for dietary supplement	Same as Day 1	Same as Day 2	Same as Day 3	Same as Day 4	Same as Day 5
Lines/Tubes/Monitors	IV fluids	Convert to saline loc		Same as Day 3	Same as Day 4	D/C saline loc
Mobility/Self-Care	*Immobile/bed rest:* TCDB q 2 h ROM q 2 h W/A Avoid positioning on ulcer, bony prominences/areas Position the patient on an angle when sidelying Use pillows under lower legs to elevate heels in supine lying and between knees and ankles when in sidelying position Use pillows or foot drop splints to position ankles to prevent contracture	Evaluate mobility level and treat as indicated		Same as Day 3	Same as Day 4	Same as Day 5

Continued

Clinical Pathway for Stage 3 Pressure Ulcer *Continued*

Aspect of Care (Cont'd)	Date_____ Day 1	Date_____ Day 2	Date_____ Day 3	Date_____ Day 4	Date_____ Day 5	Date_____ Day 6
Mobility/Self-Care (Cont'd)	*Up in chair with assistance:* TCDB q 2 h Encourage wt shifting q 2 h; if patient unable to shift wt, use pillows under ischial tuberosities Use draw sheet or bath blanket to cover chair If patient in a recliner, change its position q 1 h; use pillows under lower legs when in reclined position Patients with decreased mental status should not sit longer than 4 h *Ambulatory requiring assistance:* Assist patient with ambulation TID Reposition in bed or chair as needed *Ambulatory—independent:* Encourage ambulation QID					

Discharge Planning					
Evaluate support systems Evaluate need for preventative equipment and supplies *Discharge home:* Notify home health *Discharge NH:* Refer to case manager for NH return/referral; notify NH of pressure ulcer and treatment measures used on transfer form and in oral report	Continue as Day 1	Continue as Day 2	Evaluate progress of discharge planning and any unmet needs	Continue to resolve any problems identified on Day 4 Ensure all supplies for wound care at home	Same as Day 5

Clinical Pathway for *Stage 4 Pressure Ulcer**

ICD-9 Code **707.0**   **ELOS Length of stay is dependent upon medical condition; patient may be discharged to home or LTC facility for further treatment of the pressure ulcer**

Nursing Diagnosis/ Collaborative Problem	Expected Outcome (The Patient Is Expected to...)	Met/ Not Met	Reason	Date/ Initials
Alteration in tissue integrity	Perform wound care and understand how to prevent deterioration and further occurrence of pressure ulcers *or* If the patient is unable to, the family provides the needed care			
Pain	Be free of pain or state that pain is controlled with analgesics			

Aspect of Care	Date___ Day 1	Date___ Day 2	Date___ Day 3	Date___ Day 4	Date___ Day 5	Date___ Day 6
Assessment	Systems assessment q shift Assess skin for skin loss with muscle or bone involvement • Location • Stage • Size (include areas of redness around ulcer site)	Same as Day 1	Same as Day 2 Measure size of pressure ulcer	Same as Day 3	Same as Day 4	Same as Day 5

*Adapted with permission from Harbor Hospital Center, Baltimore, Maryland. Developed by the Interdisciplinary Wound Care Team.

• Color of wound bed • Exudate Assess need for isolation if exudate cannot be contained by dressing and signs of infection present Pressure ulcer assessment sheet x 2/week VS q 4 h Psychosocial assessment Assess for contributing factors • Immobility, inactivity • Incontinence • Malnutrition or dehydration • Frailty • Under normal wt or overwt • Diabetes • Anemia • Anascara • Immunosuppression • Systemic disease		Continue as Day 3	Continue as Day 4
			Continue as Day 5
Teaching Orient to hospital and unit Provide information concerning pressure ulcers	Continue to provide patient and family information regarding ulcer formation, prevention, and treatment	Teach patient and family dressing changes, skin care, mobility, diet	

Continued

Clinical Pathway for Stage 4 Pressure Ulcer Continued

Aspect of Care (Cont'd)	Date ___ Day 1	Date ___ Day 2	Date ___ Day 3	Date ___ Day 4	Date ___ Day 5	Date ___ Day 6
Teaching (Cont'd)	Involve family in care of patient as appropriate Review plan of care/clinical pathway with patient and family					
Consults	Dietician Enterostomal therapist Physical therapist Surgeon	N/A	N/A	N/A	N/A	N/A
Lab Tests	SMA-6(60) CBC Blood culture and gram stain Wound culture and gram stain	N/A	N/A	Blood and pressure ulcer culture	CBC, SMA-6(60)	N/A
Other Tests	ECG U/A, C & S Chest x-ray	N/A	N/A	N/A	N/A	N/A
Meds	Multivitamin QD IV/PO antibiotics if wound culture is positive and cellulitis present	Same as Day 1	Same as Day 2	Same as Day 3	Same as Day 4	Same as Day 5

Treatments/ Interventions					
Evaluate need for specialty bed using decision tree Clean wound with NS and dry skin around ulcer gently Dressing changes are placed in the order in which they should be tried • Hydroactive gel covered with gauze; if wound has necrotic tissue, change q 2 days; if wound is granulating, gel may remain up to 7 days; gel may be used with a wafer • Chlorapactin and gauze packing, change BID to TID • Algiderm wound packing for draining wounds; cover with gauze and tape and change q 1–5 days; packing may be used under a wafer Daily wt I & O	Dressing changes as needed	Same as Day 2	Remeasure and evaluate pressure ulcer Dressing change PRN	Dressing change PRN	Same as Day 5

Continued

Clinical Pathway for Stage 4 Pressure Ulcer *Continued*

Aspect of Care (Cont'd)	Date____ Day 1	Date____ Day 2	Date____ Day 3	Date____ Day 4	Date____ Day 5	Date____ Day 6
Treatments/ Interventions (Cont'd)	*Dry skin:* For bath, use mild soap or very little soap *Very dry skin:* Bath oil; apply petroleum jelly lightly to wet skin *Incontinence:* Keep skin clean and dry; use Uniwash, Unisalve (or other similar product) and/or cornstarch with each incontinent episode *Fecal incontinence:* Apply fecal pouch; evaluate need for antidiarrheals or disimpaction; use reusable underpads *Urinary incontinence:* If appropriate for males, use male external cath; change incontinent briefs when wet; do not position patient on Foley cath tubing					

Nutrition	High protein, high calorie unless contraindicted Encourage fluids Calorie count x 3 days Assess need for dietary supplement	Same as Day 1	Same as Day 2	Same as Day 3	Same as Day 4	Same as Day 5
Lines/Tubes/ Monitors	IV fluids	IV fluids	Convert to saline loc	Same as Day 3	Same as Day 4	D/C saline loc
Mobility/Self- Care	*Immobile/bed rest:* TCDB q 2 h (lift up; do not pull or drag across sheet) ROM q 2 h W/A Avoid positioning on ulcer site, bony prominences/areas Position the patient on an angle when sidelying Use pillows under lower legs to elevate heels in supine lying and between knees and ankles when in sidelying position Use pillows or foot drop splints to position ankles to prevent contracture	Evaluate mobility level and treat as indicated	Same as Day 2	Same as Day 3	Same as Day 4	Same as Day 5

Continued

Clinical Pathway for Stage 4 Pressure Ulcer Continued

Aspect of Care (Cont'd)	Date _____ Day 1	Date _____ Day 2	Date _____ Day 3	Date _____ Day 4	Date _____ Day 5	Date _____ Day 6
Mobility/Self-Care (Cont'd)	*Up in chair with assistance:* TCDB q 2 h Encourage wt shifting q 2 h; if patient unable to shift wt, use pillows under ischial tuberosities Use draw sheet or bath blanket to cover chair If patient in a recliner, change its position q 1 h; use pillows under lower legs when in reclined position Patients with decreased mental status should not sit longer than 4 h *Ambulatory requiring assistance:* Assist patient with ambulation TID Reposition in bed or chair as needed *Ambulatory— independent:* Encourage ambulation QID						

Discharge Planning					
Evaluate support systems Evaluate need for preventative equipment and supplies *Discharge home:* Notify home health *Discharge NH:* Refer to case manager for NH return/referral; notify NH of pressure ulcer and treatment measures used on transfer form and in oral report	Continue as Day 1	Continue as Day 2	Evaluate progress of discharge planning and any unmet needs	Continue to resolve any problems identified on Day 4 Ensure supplies needed are at home as applicable	Same as Day 5

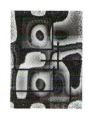

Part III

Clinical Pathways for Critical Care Patients

Unit

IX

Critical Health Problems

▼ ▼ ▼

Clinical Pathway for Complicated Myocardial Infarction

ICD-9 Code 410.91   ELOS 6 days

Nursing Diagnosis/ Collaborative Problem	Expected Outcome (The Patient Is Expected to...)	Met/ Not Met	Reason	Date/ Initials
Alteration in cardiac output	Have improved or maintained cardiac output with normal VS and a stable ECG			
Pain	State that pain is relieved or controlled with medication			
Activity intolerance	Resume ADLs with good exercise tolerance			
Anxiety and fear	Verbalize feelings about anxiety and fear and use techniques to manage these stressors			
Ineffective individual and family coping	Identify effective coping strategies			

Aspect of Care	Date____ Day 1 (ICU)	Date____ Day 2 (ICU)	Date____ Day 3 (ICU)	Date____ Day 4	Date____ Day 5	Date____ Day 6
Assessment	Systems assessment with particular attention to the cardiovascular system • Rate, rhythm, sound (S₃) • Jugular venous distention • Distal peripheral pulses • Skin temp	Same as Day 1 VS q 4 h	Same as Day 2	Systems assessment with particular attention to the cardiovascular system VS q 4 h (apical pulse) Pain assessment	Systems assessment with particular attention to the cardiovascular system VS q 4 h (apical pulse) Pain assessment	Systems assessment with particular attention to the cardiovascular system VS q shift (apical pulse)

Continued

VS q 1 h (apical pulse)	Continue to monitor for effects of meds	Continue to monitor for effects of meds
Pain assessment · Type, intensity · Duration, location · Activity when pain occurs	Continue to monitor for complications	Continue to monitor for complications
Monitor hemodynamic pressures · Pulmonary artery pressure, wedge pressure · R atrial pressure · Systemic vascular resistance · Cardiac output, CVP		
Monitor for effects of meds		
Monitor for complications · Ventricular septal rupture · CHF, PE · Bleeding secondary to thrombolytic therapy		
Psychosocial assessment		
Code status/ advance directive		

Clinical Pathway for Complicated Myocardial Infarction *Continued*

Aspect of Care (Cont'd)	Date____ Day 1 (ICU)	Date____ Day 2 (ICU)	Date____ Day 3 (ICU)	Date____ Day 4	Date____ Day 5	Date____ Day 6
Teaching	Orient to hospital and unit Prepare for diagnostic tests Provide information about diagnosis Involve family in care of patient as appropriate Review plan of care/clinical pathway with patient and family	Continue explanation of diagnosis and its relationship to stress, diet, risk factors Explain rationale for activity restrictions	Reinforce information relating to prevention of MI Teach S/S of MI and complications of an MI Begin meds instruction • Name of meds • Action/purpose • When and how to take • Side effects • What to do if dosage missed	Give healthy heart book and reinforce information about diet restrictions Information concerning resuming ADLs and exercise program If necessary provide information on wt loss, diabetes management	Assess patient's and family's understanding of previous information and reinforce as needed	Same as Day 5
Consults	Cardiologist Cardiac rehab nurse Dietician Social worker	N/A	N/A	N/A	N/A	N/A
Lab Tests	SMA-6(6/60) Cardiac enzymes, isoenzymes INR(PT)/APPT CBC with diff U/A ABGs	SMA-6(6/60) Cardiac enzymes INR(PT)/APPT CBC with diff	SMA-6(6/60) CBC with diff INR(PT)/APPT	SMA-6(6/60) INR(PT)/APPT	SMA-6(6/60)	SMA-6(6/60) CBC with diff

Other Tests	ECG ECG during acute chest pain episodes Chest x-ray Pulse ox	ECG Echocardiogram	ECG MUGA Evaluate need for stress test, cardiac cath	ECG	ECG	ECG
Meds	Thrombolytic therapy with TPA or streptokinase Vasodilator (nitroglycerin) Beta blockers (propranolol) Calcium channel blockers (diltiazem) Antiaggregants (ASA) Analgesic for pain (morphine) Sedatives (lorazepam) may be used for anxiety and/or sleep Stool softener	Nitroglycerin Beta blockers Calcium channel blockers Anticoagulant Antiaggregants Analgesic for pain Stool softener	Same as Day 2 Change to PO meds for pain	Same as Day 3 Assess need to D/C anticoagulant	Same as Day 4	Same as Day 5
Treatments/ Interventions	Continuous cardiac monitoring O₂ per NC if hypoxic Strict I & O Daily wt ROM q 4 h W/A	Same as Day 1	Same as Day 2	Transfer to telemetry unit Cardiac monitoring I & O Daily wt	Same as Day 4	D/C I & O and daily wts, if no evidence of failure

Continued

Clinical Pathway for Complicated Myocardial Infarction *Continued*

Aspect of Care (Cont'd)	Date____ Day 1 (ICU)	Date____ Day 2 (ICU)	Date____ Day 3 (ICU)	Date____ Day 4	Date____ Day 5	Date____ Day 6
Nutrition	NPO	Liquids or a low fat, low cholesterol and low sodium No iced beverages No caffeine Fluid restriction	Same as Day 2	Low fat, low sodium, low cholesterol	Same as Day 4	Same as Day 5
Lines/Tubes/Monitors	IV fluids Triple lumen cath Intra-aortic balloon pump (IAPB)	Same as Day 1 May D/C IAPB	IV fluids Discontinue IAPB	Convert IV to saline loc	Same as Day 4	D/C saline loc
Mobility/Self-Care	Bed rest Assist with ADLs	Bed rest	Up in chair TID	Same as Day 3	Ambulate in room TID	Ambulate in hall QID
Discharge Planning	Assess need for social services, financial status, health insurance and coverage, home environment, need for placement, and family support	Continue as on Day 1 Interview family regarding home situation and need for changes or modifications in the home	Refer to cardiac rehab program	Refer to the American Heart Association and local support groups	Support family as needed with home modifications and adaptive/assistive devices if needed	Arrange for • Follow-up visit with MD • Home health nurse visit • Cardiac rehab nurse

Notes

Clinical Pathway for Percutaneous Transluminal Coronary Angioplasty (PTCA)

ICD-9 Code 414   **ELOS 3 days**

Nursing Diagnosis/ Collaborative Problem	Expected Outcome (The Patient Is Expected to...)	Met/ Not Met	Reason	Date/ Initials
Anxiety	Verbalize fears and ask questions regarding diagnosis and treatment			
Pain	State that pain is relieved with medication			
Activity intolerance	Resume ADLs with good exercise tolerance			

Aspect of Care	Date____ Pre-procedure	Date____ Day 1	Date____ Day 2	Date____ Day 3
Assessment	Systems assessment with attention to cardiovascular system • Rate, rhythm, sounds • Capillary refill • Pulses Pain assessment VS q 4 h Psychosocial assessment Pre-op check list	*Recovery area/PACU:* VS q 15 min x 4, then q 30 min x 4 Check groin for bleeding Check distal pulses Systems and pain assessment *Post-procedure:* VS q 1 h x 4, then q 4 h Systems and pain assessment	Systems assessment Pain assessment VS q 4 h Check groin for bleeding Check for distal pulses Continue to monitor for complications	Same as Day 2

Teaching	Orient to hospital and unit Reinforce information about procedure • Cardiac cath lab • Where cath inserted • Sensations during procedure • What to tell MD during procedure • Meds used during procedure (heparin, nitroglycerin) Involve family in care of patient as appropriate Review plan of care/clinical pathway with patient and family	Check groin for bleeding Check pulses Monitor for complications • Bleeding • Diminished or absent pulses • Increased chest pain Continue to reinforce information about diagnosis • Notify nurse of chest pain or discomfort Provide information about discharge meds	Reinforce Day 1	Reinforce information concerning diet, exercise, activity, and meds
Consults	Cardiology Anesthesia clearance (standby) Cardiac surgeon (standby)	Dietician	N/A	N/A

Continued

Clinical Pathway for Percutaneous Transluminal Coronary Angioplasty (PTCA) *Continued*

Aspect of Care (Cont'd)	Date ___ Pre-procedure	Date ___ Day 1	Date ___ Day 2	Date ___ Day 3
Lab Tests	CBC with diff SMA-12 U/A Type and hold 4 units of blood INR(PT)/APTT	INR(PT)/APTT Hgb and Hct	INR(PT)/APTT	N/A
Other Tests	Chest x-ray ECG Be sure cardiac cath films available	N/A	N/A	N/A
Meds	Prednisone PO at bedtime Calcium channel blocker Heparin	Continuous heparin drip	D/C heparin drip	N/A
Treatments/ Interventions	Cardiac monitor O₂ PRN I & O	Cardiac monitor Keep involved leg immobilized with sandbag to insertion site D/C sandbag 6–8 h after procedure completed, if bleeding stopped O₂ PRN I & O	Cardiac monitor I & O	Same as Day 2

Nutrition	NPO pre-procedure	Low Na$^+$ and cholesterol diet Encourage fluids unless restricted	Same as Day 2	Same as Day 3
Lines/Tubes/Monitors	Saline loc	Continuous IV fluids ($\frac{1}{2}$NS)	D/C IV fluids	N/A
Mobility/Self-Care	As tolerated	Strict bed rest Turn with assistance HOB elevated 15–30°	Up in chair and ambulate as tolerated	Same as Day 3
Discharge Planning	Assess need for social services, financial status, health insurance and coverage, home environment, and family support	Discuss work restrictions and potential financial implications Discuss home modifications, if needed Arrange for supplies and equipment, if needed	Arrange for follow-up appointment with MD Ensure that needed equipment at home in time for discharge	Same as Day 3

Clinical Pathway for Coronary Artery Bypass Graft (CABG) (Without Cardiac Catheterization)

ICD-9 Code **36.10**   ELOS **7 days**

Nursing Diagnosis/ Collaborative Problem	Expected Outcome (The Patient Is Expected to...)	Met/ Not Met	Reason	Date/ Initials
High risk for decreased cardiac output	Have heart rate <120, BP >100 mm Hg, no dysrhythmias, and no complaints of chest discomfort/pain; O$_2$ saturation >90%			
Potential for postoperative complications (infection, F & E imbalance, hypotension or hypertension, hypothermia, cardiac tamponade)	Have Hgb and Hct WNL, WBC WNL, clean and dry incision, VS within baseline, no S/S of F & E imbalance			
Pain (incisional)	State that surgical pain is reduced or alleviated following appropriate interventions			
Activity intolerance	Ambulate in hall ad lib without fatigue or dyspnea			
Altered health/home maintenance	Follow recommendations for lifelong changes in lifestyle			

Aspect of Care	Date _____ Pre-admission/ Pre-op	Date _____ Day 1 (DOS) (ICU)	Date _____ Day 2 (POD #1) (ICU → telemetry)	Date _____ Day 3 (POD #2)	Date _____ Day 4 (POD #3)	Date _____ Day 5 (POD #4)	Date _____ Day 6 (POD #5)	Date _____ Day 7 (POD #6)
Assessment	Systems assessment with focus on cardiovascular assessment Pre-op checklist Psychosocial assessment	Systems assessment VS 15 min x 2 h, then q 1–2 h, depending on stability Assess patient tolerance to weaning off ventilator 6–24 h post-op Pain assessment Hemodynamic monitoring Check dressings for intactness and drainage Check wound drain(s) Check chest tube system	VS q 2–4 h, depending on stability Hemodynamic monitoring Systems assessment with primary focus on cardiovascular/ respiratory assessments Check dressings and drains when doing VS Check chest tube system until D/C'd Pulse ox after arterial line D/C'd	Systems assessment with focus on cardiovascular assessment Check on BM Pulse ox VS q 4 h Monitor incisions for drainage, S/S of infection	Same as Day 3	Systems assessment VS q 4 h Assess incisions	Systems assessment VS QID Assess incisions	Same as Day 6
Teaching	Review clinical pathway/plan of care with patient and family	Reinforce post-op expectations and course with family	Teach about transfer to step-down unit/ telemetry	Review activity progression Review diet restrictions, including ↓ caffeine	Continue with discharge teaching regarding • Diet • Meds • Wound care	Same as Day 4	Continue with discharge teaching; provide verbal and written instructions	Same as Day 6

Continued

Clinical Pathway for CABG (Without Cardiac Catheterization) Continued

Aspect of Care (Cont'd)	Date ___ Pre-admission/ Pre-op	Date ___ Day 1 (DOS) (ICU)	Date ___ Day 2 (POD #1) (ICU → telemetry)	Date ___ Day 3 (POD #2)	Date ___ Day 4 (POD #3)	Date ___ Day 5 (POD #4)	Date ___ Day 6 (POD #5)	Date ___ Day 7 (POD #6)
Teaching (Cont'd)	Teach importance of strictly following pre-op instructions regarding meds (such as D/C'ing diuretics, aspirin, anticoagulants, and digoxin before surgery as MD specified) Reinforce nature of surgery and post-op expectations, such as chest tubes, endotracheal tube with ventilator, Foley, IVs, pain management, incisions, DB & C, incentive spirometer		Reinforce need and procedures for DB & C/ incentive spirometer	Begin teaching on postdischarge activity, meds, wound care	• Activity progression/ restrictions • Sexual activity • Post-op complications • S/S to report to MD • Cardiac rehab			
Consults	Cardiology	Respiratory therapy	Social worker Cardiac rehab	Dietitian for teaching	N/A	N/A	N/A	N/A

Lab Tests	Admission lab work, including CBC with diff, SMA-6 (6/60), INR(PT)/APTT, type and cross match or screen, Cr	ABGs q 4 h x 12 h, SMA-6 (6/60), CPK, Hgb and Hct x 2	ABG Hbg and Hct CPK SMA-6 (6/60)	N/A	N/A	CBC, SMA-6 (6/60)	N/A	N/A
Other Tests	ECG Chest x-ray	ECG Chest x-ray	Same as Day 1	N/A	N/A	ECG Chest x-ray	N/A	N/A
Meds	Cardiac meds as MD specified; Pre-anesthesia meds; Prophylactic antibiotic at least 1 h before OR	IV antibiotic q 6–8 h x 48 h; Zantac 150 mg BID; ASA; IV or IM morphine PRN; Vasoactive meds as needed	Same as Day 1 plus cardiac meds as appropriate, K+ supplement, diuretic, heparin SQ q 8 h	D/C antibiotics; Pain med (IV, IM, or PO) PRN; Cardiac meds as appropriate; ASA; Heparin; Zantac; Stool softener at bedtime	Pain med PRN; Cardiac meds; ASA; Heparin; Zantac; Stool softener at bedtime; Laxative of choice PRN	D/C Zantac, heparin; ASA; Cardiac meds; Stool softener at bedtime; Laxative of choice PRN	ASA; Cardiac meds as appropriate; Stool softener at bedtime	Same as Day 6
Treatments/ Interventions	Provide emotional support	I & O q h → q 2 h; Ventilator/wean; Supplemental oxygen after extubation; Incentive spirometer q h W/A; Antiembolism stockings	Transfer to telemetry or step-down unit; O₂ via NC per pulse ox readings; Daily wt; I & O q 8 h; Elevate operative leg	Telemetry; O₂ via NC PRN; Daily wt; Antiembolism stockings; Pacer wires	Telemetry; O₂ PRN; Daily wt; Antiembolism stockings; Pacer wires; Provide emotional support	Same as Day 4	Telemetry; D/C pacer wires; Incisional care; Continue with emotional support; Daily wt	Telemetry; Remove staples/sutures; Incisional care; Psychosocial support; Daily wt

Continued

Clinical Pathway for CABG (Without Cardiac Catheterization) *Continued*

Aspect of Care (Cont'd)	Date ___ Pre-admission/ Pre-op	Date ___ Day 1 (DOS) (ICU)	Date ___ Day 2 (POD #1) (ICU → telemetry)	Date ___ Day 3 (POD #2)	Date ___ Day 4 (POD #3)	Date ___ Day 5 (POD #4)	Date ___ Day 6 (POD #5)	Date ___ Day 7 (POD #6)
Treatments/ Interventions (Cont'd)		SCDs Pacer wires Elevate operative leg	Pacer wires Antiembolism stockings	Provide emotional support MD to remove/ change surgical dressings	Incisional care			
Nutrition	Low cholesterol/ low sodium Caffeine free NPO after 12 midnight	NPO	Clear liquids if BS present	Advance DAT (low cholesterol/ low sodium, caffeine free)	DAT	Same as Day 4	Same as Day 5	Same as Day 6
Lines/Tubes/ Monitors	N/A	Continuous IV fluids (Lactated Ringer's → 5% D/$\frac{1}{2}$NS) (peripheral/central) Foley cath Arterial line PA line NGT CVP line Continuous cardiac monitoring Autotransfusion Chest tubes	D/C Foley in AM D/C IV when adequate PO intake; convert to saline loc D/C arterial line, PA line, NGT (may clamp to determine tolerance before removal), CVP Cardiac monitor D/C chest tubes D/C autotransfusion	Cardiac monitor Saline loc	Same as Day 3	Same as Day 4	Same as Day 5	D/C saline loc and cardiac monitor

Mobility/ Self-Care	As tolerated	Bed rest Turn q 2 h after hemodynamically stable HOB ↑ at least 30°	Dangle after extubation OOB to chair once if tolerated dangling HOB ↑	BRPs with assistance x 2–4/day OOB in chair TID	Ambulate into hall 50–100 feet x 4–6/day	Ambulate into hall 100–200 feet x 6/day	Ambulate ad lib	Same as Day 6
Discharge Planning	N/A	Begin to assess personal support systems and home care situation	Continue with Day 1	Assess ability for home care and need for home health services	Arrange for follow-up by home health services if needed for home discharge	Continue with Day 4	Refer to American Heart Association for further support/information Arrange for follow-up through cardiac rehab department	Make follow-up appointment as MD specified

Clinical Pathway for Thoractomy (for Lung Cancer)

ICD-9 Code 162.9/34.02   ELOS 6 days

Nursing Diagnosis/Collaborative Problem	Expected Outcome (The Patient Is Expected to...)	Met/Not Met	Reason	Date/Initials
Impaired gas exchange	Have no adventitious breath sounds, ABGs WNL, and pulse ox >90%; breathe without dyspnea			
Pain	State that pain is alleviated or minimized following appropriate interventions			
Potential for postoperative complications (hemorrhage, infection, mediastinal shift)	Have Hgb and Hct WNL, WBC WNL, incision clean and dry			
Body image disturbance/ineffective coping	Verbalize feelings about loss of all or part of lung; identify coping mechanisms that have been used in the past			

Aspect of Care	Date_____ Pre-admission/Pre-op	Date_____ Day 1 (DOS)	Date_____ Day 2 (POD #1)	Date_____ Day 3 (POD #2)	Date_____ Day 4 (POD #3)	Date_____ Day 5–6 (POD #4–5)
Assessment	Systems assessment Pre-op checklist Psychosocial assessment	*PACU:* VS q 15 min x 4, q 30 min x 4, then q 1 h Monitor chest tube drainage system Systems assessment with focus on respiratory assessment	VS q 2–4 h (depending on stability) Respiratory assessment q 2 h Pain assessment Pulse ox	VS q 4 h with respiratory assessment Pain assessment Monitor chest tube drainage system Monitor incision for drainage and intactness	VS q 4 h with respiratory assessment Monitor incision for drainage and intactness Pain assessment	Same as Day 4

		Pain assessment; Check surgical dressing and drains; *Post-op:* VS q 1 h x 4; if stable, VS q 2 h with respiratory assessments; Systems assessment; Pain assessment; Pulse ox; Check surgical dressing and drains; Monitor chest tube drainage system	Check surgical dressing and drains; Monitor chest tube drainage system; Check for spontaneous voiding after Foley out; Check bowel sounds; Systems assessment	Systems assessment; Assess for BM	Systems assessment	
Teaching	Review clinical pathway/plan of care with patient and family; Reinforce nature of surgery and post-op expectations, including chest tubes, pain management, respiratory treatments, and possible adjunct treatment with radiation or chemotherapy	Orient to hospital and unit; Review post-op expectations, including instruction on DB & C and incentive spirometer; Teach patient to report unusual S/S, including difficulty in breathing or severe pain	Same as Day 1	Same as Day 2	Begin discharge teaching regarding • Pain management • Wound care • Activity restrictions • Post-op complications • S/S to report to MD • Meds	Review discharge instructions per Day 4
Consults	Oncology	Respiratory therapy	Social worker	N/A	N/A	N/A

Continued

Clinical Pathway for Thoractomy (for Lung Cancer) Continued

Aspect of Care (Cont'd)	Date ___ Pre-admission/ Pre-op	Date ___ Day 1 (DOS)	Date ___ Day 2 (POD #1)	Date ___ Day 3 (POD #2)	Date ___ Day 4 (POD #3)	Date ___ Day 5–6 (POD #4–5)
Lab Tests	Admission labs, including CBC with diff, SMA-6 (6/60), Cr, ABGs, PT(INR)/APTT	CBC, lytes	CBC, lytes	Hgb and Hct in AM	Same as Day 3	Same as Day 4
Other Tests	ECG Chest x-ray Pulmonary function tests Ventilation/ perfusion scan	Chest x-ray	Same as Day 1	Same as Day 2	Same as Day 3	N/A
Meds	Pre-anesthesia meds Pre-op prophylactic antibiotic at least 1 h before OR	PCA or IM morphine or meperidine Antibiotics IVPB q 6–8 h x 48 h Tylenol suppository for ↑temp PRN Antiemetic IV push or IM PRN	IM pain med; D/C PCA Continue with antibiotics Tylenol suppository for ↑temp PRN Antiemetic PRN	IM or PO analgesic PRN Stool softener at bedtime	PO analgesic PRN Stool softener at bedtime Laxative of choice PRN	Same as Day 4
Treatments/ Interventions	N/A	O₂ per mask or NC DB & C with incentive spirometer q 1–2 h Antiembolism stockings SCDs/Venodynes I & O q 2–4 h	Respiratory treatments with nebulizer or IPPB, if smoker or history of recent smoking O₂ per NC if pulse ox <90% DB & C with incentive spirometer q 1–2 h	MD to remove/ change surgical dressing and wound drain(s) DB & C/incentive spirometer q 2 h W/A Antiembolism stockings	Keep stab wound(s) covered with dry sterile dressing DB & C/incentive spirometer q 2 h W/A Antiembolism stockings	Change stab wound dressings QD and PRN DB & C/incentive spirometer q 2 h W/A Antiembolism stockings

		SCDs/Venodynes Antiembolism stockings I & O q 8 h	Respiratory treatments if smoker or history of recent smoking		
Nutrition	NPO after 12 midnight	NPO	Begin clear liquids → advance as tolerated	DAT	Same as Day 3	Same as Day 4
Lines/Tubes/ Monitors	N/A	Continuous IV fluids with KCl (Lactated Ringer's → 5% D$\frac{1}{2}$NS) Foley cath Chest tube(s) to wall suction Wound drain(s)	Convert IV to saline loc if voiding and no nausea D/C Foley Chest tube(s) to wall suction Wound drain(s)	Chest tube(s) to wall suction	MD to remove chest tube(s)	N/A
Mobility/Self-Care	Up ad lib	Bed rest Turn q 2 h; do not turn onto operative side	Up in chair BID with assistance Assist with ADLs as needed Leg exercises, such as quad sets and ankle pumps, q 2 h Assist with turning as needed	Up in room with supervision/assistance TID Continue with leg exercises while in bed	Up in room with supervision ad lib Continue with leg exercises while in bed	Ambulate in hall ad lib May shower per MD protocol
Discharge Planning	N/A	Assess home environment for support systems	Same as Day 1	Assess need for placement if unable to return home	If discharged to home, make arrangements for home health services and necessary equipment If need for discharge to LTC facility, arrange for transfer	Refer to American Cancer Society/ American Lung Association Make follow-up appointment as MD specified

Clinical Pathway for Pulmonary Embolism (Without Mechanical Ventilation)

ICD-9 Code 415.1   ELOS 7 days

Nursing Diagnosis/ Collaborative Problem	Expected Outcome (The Patient Is Expected to…)	Met/ Not Met	Reason	Date/ Initials
Pain (chest)	State that pain is minimized following appropriate interventions			
Dyspnea, possible crackles	Have respiratory rate return to baseline; have no adventitious sounds; O_2 saturation >90%			
Potential for cardiac complications, such as dysrhythmias, abnormal ECG	Have normal sinus rhythm, pulse rate and quality return to baseline, and no S_3 or S_4 heart sounds present			
Anxiety and fear	Verbalize feelings regarding condition, especially dyspnea and chest pain			

Aspect of Care	Date____ Day 1	Date____ Day 2	Date____ Day 3	Date____ Day 4	Date____ Day 5	Date____ Day 6–7
Assessment	Systems assessment Chest pain assessment and respiratory assessment q 1–2 h Pulse ox	Same as Day 1	VS q 4 h with respiratory assessment Pulse ox Systems assessment	Same as Day 3	Same as Day 4	Same as Day 5

VS q 1–2 h, depending on severity of condition Assess for cardiac complications Assess for bleeding tendencies		Assess for bleeding tendencies			
Teaching Orient to hospital and unit routines Review clinical pathway/plan of care with patient and family Review diagnosis and answer questions	Same as Day 1	Teach measures to help prevent further thrombo-embolitic complications, such as ↑ mobility, wt loss, no oral contraceptives Teach early S/S of DVT	Review teaching from Day 3	Begin discharge teaching regarding • Anticoagulation therapy • Bleeding precautions • Need for follow-up lab work/diagnostic tests • Activity restrictions • Reduction of risk factors • S/S to report to MD	Reinforce discharge instructions (verbal and written)
Consults Surgery (if indicated) Respiratory therapy	Dietitian, if indicated for weight reduction	N/A	N/A	N/A	N/A
Lab Tests CBC with diff, SMA-6 (6/60), INR(PT)/APTT, ABGs	INR(PT)/APTT	INR(PT)/APTT ABGs	INR(PT)/APTT	Same as Day 4	Same as Day 5

Continued

Clinical Pathway for Pulmonary Embolism (Without Mechanical Ventilation) *Continued*

Aspect of Care (Cont'd)	Date ___ Day 1	Date ___ Day 2	Date ___ Day 3	Date ___ Day 4	Date ___ Day 5	Date ___ Day 6-7
Other Tests	ECG Chest x-ray Ventilation/ perfusion scan Vascular studies (if DVT suspected) Pulmonary angiography (for nonconclusive ventilation/ perfusion scan)	ECG	Same as Day 2	N/A	N/A	N/A
Meds	Continuous IV heparin via electronic device Stool softener QD PO analgesic PRN	Same as Day 1	Continuous IV heparin Start on oral anticoagulant (Coumadin) Stool softener QD PO analgesic PRN	Continuous IV heparin at ↓ rate Coumadin dose based on lab values Stool softener PO analgesic PRN	Same as Day 4 (continue decreasing heparin rate per MD)	Same as Day 5
Treatments/ Interventions	I & O q 8 h Oxygen via N/C or mask Antiembolism stockings SCDs or Venodynes Emotional support Incentive spirom- eter q 2 h W/A	Same as Day 1	Same as Day 2	D/C I & O O$_2$ PRN Antiembolism stockings SCDs or Venodynes Incentive spirom- eter q 2 h W/A	Same as Day 4	Same as Day 5

	Day 1	Day 2	Day 3	Day 4	Day 5	Day 6
Nutrition	DAT (unless need for calorie/fat restriction)	Same as Day 1	Same as Day 2	Same as Day 3	Same as Day 4	Same as Day 5
Lines/Tubes/ Monitors	Cardiac monitoring Continous IV fluids at low rate	Same as Day 1 Convert IV to saline loc if adequate PO fluids	D/C cardiac monitor Saline loc	Saline loc	Same as Day 4	D/C saline loc
Mobility/Self-Care	Bed rest HOB up at least 30° Leg exercises, such as ROM, quad sets, ankle pumps, q 2 h, *unless* DVT in LE If DVT suspected, elevate affected LE Assist with ADLs as needed	Same as Day 1	Same as Day 2	Up in chair BID with assistance as needed While in bed, keep HOB ↑ to 30° or higher Leg exercises q 2 h W/A If DVT, remain on bed rest with affected leg elevated Assist with ADLs as needed	Up in room ad lib unless DVT present Leg exercises while in bed	Up in hall ad lib unless DVT present Leg exercises while in bed
Discharge Planning	Assess home environment and personal support systems	Same as Day 1	Same as Day 2	Assess need for placement if patient unable to go home	Arrange for follow-up home health services if needed Arrange for transfer to LTC or other facility if needed	Arrange for follow-up appointment as MD specified Provide information for patient about lab services and availability

Clinical Pathway for Head Injury*

ICD-9 Code 854   ELOS 7 days

Nursing Diagnosis/ Collaborative Problem	Expected Outcome (The Patient Is Expected to...)	Met/ Not Met	Reason	Date/ Initials
Altered cerebral tissue perfusion	Maintain baseline vital and neuro signs			
Sensory perceptual alteration	Regain sensory and cognitive awareness			
Ineffective airway clearance, impaired gas exchange, ineffective breathing pattern	Maintain a patent airway and normal ABGs			
Impaired physical mobility	Remain free of complications of immobility			
Self-care deficit	Performs some self-care activities with assistive/ adaptive devices			
Impaired verbal communication	Utilize communication strategies via speaking, communication board, or voice synthesizer			
Ineffective family coping	The family will verbalize understanding of the patient's injury and will begin to adjust to the changes in the patient's physical and cognitive status			

*This pathway is a general guideline and must be modified for severity of injury.

Aspect of Care	Date ___ Day 1 (ICU)	Date ___ Day 2 (ICU)	Date ___ Day 3 (ICU)	Date ___ Day 4	Date ___ Day 5	Date ___ Day 6	Date ___ Day 7
Assessment	Systems assessment with attention to neuro and respiratory system • Eye, motor, and verbal response • LOC, pupils • Cranial nerves • Cognitive and language deficit • Respiratory rate, rhythm VS and neuro signs q 1 h Cardiac monitor Ventilator settings Monitor for complications • Cerebral edema • Hematoma • SIADH • Hydrocephalus • Seizures • CSF leak • Stress ulcers • Meningitis Psychosocial assessment	Same as Day 1	Same as Day 2 except VS and neuro checks q 2 h D/C ventilator checks	Same as Day 3 except VS and neuro checks q 4 h	Same as Day 4	Same as Day 5	VS and neuro checks q 8 h

Continued

Clinical Pathway for Head Injury *Continued*

Aspect of Care	Date_____ Day 1 (ICU)	Date_____ Day 2 (ICU)	Date_____ Day 3 (ICU)	Date_____ Day 4	Date_____ Day 5	Date_____ Day 6	Date_____ Day 7
Teaching	Orient to unit and hospital Prepare for diagnostic tests Provide information about diagnosis Involve family in care of patient as appropriate Review care plan/clinical pathway with patient and/or family	Prepare for diagnostic tests Continue education regarding diagnosis and prognosis Prepare family for changes in patient's cognitive abilities Continue family involvement	Same as Day 2 Teach family ROM, sensory stimulation techniques Prepare for transfer out of ICU	Orient to unit Involve family as appropriate Bowel and bladder training program per protocol	Same as Day 4 Provide information about diagnosis and treatment Swallowing program ADLs training	Same as Day 5 Reinforce information about how to handle issues related to cognitive deficits	Same as Day 6
Consults	Dietician Respiratory therapy Social worker	Rehab services: PT/OT/SLP Swallowing evaluation	N/A	N/A	N/A	N/A	N/A
Lab Tests	CBC with diff SMA-6 (6/60) Coag studies Drug and alcohol screen ABGs U/A	Serum albumin, total protein CBC SMA-6 (6/60) ABGs	CBC SMA-6 (6/60)	CBC SMA-6 (6/60)	CBC, SMA-6 (6/60), protein, albumin	N/A	N/A

Other Tests	CT scan or MRI Skull x-ray C-spine Chest x-ray ECG	N/A	N/A	N/A	N/A	N/A	N/A
Meds	Diuretics such as mannitol or furosemide Anticonvulsant H$_2$ blocker Acetaminophen for fever >101°	Same as Day 1	D/C osmotic diuretic Anticonvulsant H$_2$ blocker	Same as Day 3 Acetaminophen for headache or fever >101°	Same as Day 4	Same as Day 5	Same as Day 6
Treatments/ Interventions	Strict I & O Urine specific gravity and osmolality q 1 h Endotracheal tube care Elevate HOB 30° to 45° Seizure precautions Suction PRN Thigh-high antiembolism stockings Daily wts Mouth care q shift Quiet environment Prevent from injury	Same as Day 1	Same as Day 2 except D/C endotracheal tube care D/C urine specific gravity, etc.	Strict I & O Elevate HOB 30° to 45° Seizure precautions Suction PRN Thigh-high antiembolism stockings Daily wts Mouth care q shift Quiet environment Prevent from injury Swallowing evaluation	I & O Thigh-high antiembolism stockings	Same as Day 5	Same as Day 5

Continued

Clinical Pathway for Head Injury *Continued*

Aspect of Care	Date_____ Day 1 (ICU)	Date_____ Day 2 (ICU)	Date_____ Day 3 (ICU)	Date_____ Day 4	Date_____ Day 5	Date_____ Day 6	Date_____ Day 7
Nutrition	NPO	Begin tube feedings or hyperalimenation	Same as Day 2	Same as Day 3 Calorie count Begin PO fluids and advance DAT based on swallowing evaluation and bowel sounds present	Mechanical soft diet	Same as Day 5	Soft diet
Lines/Tubes/ Monitors	Continuous IV fluids via triple lumen cath Ventilator Foley NGT	Same as Day 1	D/C ventilator D/C Foley D/C triple lumen and insert saline loc	IV to saline loc	Same as Day 4	D/C saline loc	N/A
Mobility/Self-Care	Bed rest TCDB q 2 h ROM to all extremities q 4 h Maintain body alignment and support extremities with pillows, minimize stress on joints Use footboard, boots to prevent foot drop	Same as Day 1	Same as Day 2 except OOB BID	Same as Day 3 OOB TID	OOB QID Begin gait training	Same as Day 5	Same as Day 6

Discharge Planning						
Social worker to assess need for social services, financial status, health insurance and coverage, home environment, need for placement, and family support	Same as Day 1	Identify placement for discharge • Rehab • ECF • Home	Begin discharge instruction and notes for transfer *or* Ensure that home equipped with assistive/adaptive devices and family/patient know how to use	Continue as Day 4 Refer to local and national head injury association Prepare for transfer to rehab or ECF	Arrange transportation Ensure transfer notes and patient care plan written	Provide family support

Clinical Pathway for Hyperglycemic Hyperosmolar Nonketotic Coma (HHNC)

ICD-9 Code 250.23 **ELOS 3 days**

Nursing Diagnosis/ Collaborative Problem	Expected Outcome (The Patient Is Expected to...)	Met/ Not Met	Reason	Date/ Initials
Fluid volume deficit	Return to appropriate fluid balance for usual state of health			
Altered nutritional status	Eat a balanced diet and maintain blood sugar and electrolytes WNL			
High risk for injury	Remain free from injury			

Aspect of Care	Date_____ Day 1	Date_____ Day 2	Date_____ Day 3
Assessment	Systems assessment VS and neuro checks q 1 h until stable, then q 4 h Monitor for S/S of dehydration, lethargy, shock Assess for underlying cause: sepsis, MI, infection Review medical history for diuretics, steroids, phenytoin Psychosocial assessment	Same as Day 1	Same as Day 2

Teaching	Orient to hospital and unit / Prepare for diagnostic tests / Provide information about diagnosis / Involve family in care of patient as appropriate / Review plan of care/clinical pathway with patient and family	Teach the patient how to avoid dehydration / Reinforce blood glucose monitoring (FSBS) / Discuss causes of HHNC	Same as Day 2
Consults	Dietician / Endocrinologist / Social worker	N/A	N/A
Lab Tests	Lytes, glucose, bicarb q 4 h / Plasma ketones, osmolarity, free fatty acids / Urine for glucose, osmolarity / ABGs / CBC	Lytes and glucose AM and PM	Lytes and glucose
Other Tests	Chest x-ray / ECG	N/A	N/A
Meds	Regular insulin bolus over q 30–60 min until glucose stable (avoid rapid decrease in serum glucose) / Sulfonylurea (Dymelor, Diabinese, Tolinase) / IV K+ and phosphate replacement	Sulfonylurea agents	Same as Day 2

Continued

Clinical Pathway for Hyperglycemic Hyperosmolar Nonketotic Coma (HHNC) Continued

Aspect of Care (Cont'd)	Date_____ Day 1	Date_____ Day 2	Date_____ Day 3
Treatments/Interventions	Strict I & O; urine specific gravity with each voiding Blood glucose q 1 h; urine for ketones each void Seizure precautions Mouth care q 2 h ROM Daily wts	I & O Urine specific gravity with each voiding Daily wts Seizure precautions	Same as Day 2
Nutrition	Encourage fluids, ice chips ADA diet	ADA diet	Same as Day 2
Lines/Tubes/Monitors	1000–2000 mL NS IV x 2–4 h Maintenance IV 0.45 NS (rate determined by wt, output, presence pulmonary/cardiac/renal problems) Change IV to 5%D/W or 5%D/NS when glucose <300	Continue IV fluids of 5%D/0.45 NS at KVO	D/C IV fluids
Mobility/Self-Care	Bed rest	OOB and ambulate as tolerated	Same as Day 2
Discharge Planning	Assess need for social services, financial status, health insurance and coverage, home environment, need for placement and family support	Continue as Day 1	Arrange for follow-up visit with MD

Notes

Clinical Pathway for Ventilator Dependency: Weaning*

ICD-9 Code 518.81   ELOS 7–30 days depending on current and pre-existing medical condition

Nursing Diagnosis/ Collaborative Problem	Expected Outcome (The Patient Is Expected to...)	Met/ Not Met	Reason	Date/ Initials
Impaired gas exchange and ineffective breathing pattern	Be weaned from the ventilator; return to baseline respiratory rate; have no adventitious sounds			
Anxiety and fear	Verbalize fears about weaning process and use stress reduction techniques to manage anxiety			

Aspect of Care	Date ___ Day 1	Date ___ Day 2	Date ___ Day 3	Date ___ Day 4	Date ___ Day 5	Date ___ Day 6	Date ___ Day 7 →
Assessment	Systems assessment with focus on respiratory and cardiac systems • Breath/lung sounds • Spontaneous respirations • Ventilator settings • Heart rate and rhythm • BP VS 4 h Pulse ox Nutrition	Same as Day 1	Same as Day 2	Same as Day 3	Same as Day 4	Same as Day 5	Same as Day 6

*These are general guidelines for the medically stable patient.

Continued

Skin assessment Sleep/rest pattern Readiness to wean • Respiratory rate • Tidal volume • Minute ventilation • Maximum volume ventilation • Vital capacity • Negative inspiratory force • Dead space ventilation • Need to insert tracheal tube or increase size of endotracheal tube Prior to weaning trial • VS • Cardiac rhythm • ABGs result or pulse ox • Anxiety • Patient/family understanding	Readiness to wean • Respiratory rate • Tidal volume • Minute ventilation • Maximum volume ventilation • Vital capacity • Negative inspiratory force • Dead space ventilation Prior to weaning trial • VS • Cardiac rhythm • Pulse ox • Anxiety • Patient/family understanding

Clinical Pathway for Ventilator Dependency: Weaning *Continued*

Aspect of Care (Cont'd)	Date ____ Day 1	Date ____ Day 2	Date ____ Day 3	Date ____ Day 4	Date ____ Day 5	Date ____ Day 6	Date ____ Day 7 →
Assessment (Cont'd)	Monitor for indications to stop weaning trial • VS changes • PVCs • Decreased LOC • Increased anxiety Monitor for complications • Fever • Malnutrition • Anemia • Pneumonia	Same as Day 1					
Teaching	Involve patient and family in developing planning care Review plan of care/clinical pathway with patient and family Explain weaning procedure • Why and how • Staff role • Patient/ family role	Reinforce Day 1 information Relaxation techniques • Guided imagery • Biofeedback	Same as Day 2	Diet, exercise Weaning program	Same as Day 4	Same as Day 5	Prepare for ventilator to be D/C'd Teach breathing exercises

	Develop daily care and weaning schedule with patient and post in room • Therapies/tests • ADLs/patient care • Weaning times • Rest periods Provide information about diet and exercises						
Consults	Dietician Pulmonologist Rehab services Respiratory therapist Social services	Same as Day 1	N/A	N/A	N/A	N/A	N/A
Lab Tests	ABGs SMA-6 (6/60) CBC Finger stick q 6 h, if on TPN	ABGs SMA-6 (6/60) FSBS, if on TPN	Same as Day 2 Hgb and Hct	N/A	Hgb and Hct ABGs	N/A	SMA-6 (6/60) Hgb and Hct ABGs
Other Tests	Chest x-ray	N/A	N/A	Chest x-ray	N/A	N/A	Chest x-ray

Continued

Clinical Pathway for Ventilator Dependency: Weaning *Continued*

Aspect of Care (Cont'd)	Date ___ Day 1	Date ___ Day 2	Date ___ Day 3	Date ___ Day 4	Date ___ Day 5	Date ___ Day 6	Date ___ Day 7 →
Meds	Bronchodilators: beta₂ agonist Inhaled cortico-steroids for inflammation Other meds as determined by medical condition	Same as Day 1	Same as Day 2	Same as Day 3 D/C cortico-steroids	Same as Day 4	Same as Day 5	D/C broncho-dilators Meds as deter-mined by medical condition
Treatments/ Interventions	Correct under-lying medical problems Strict I & O Wt QOD Incentive spirometry Pulmonary hygiene: • TCDB • Suction PRN • Chest physiotherapy • Hydration Weaning trial • Follow protocol • Initial 5–10 min trial q 3 h W/A • Provide diversional activities • Stay with patient	Same as Day 1 except • Weaning trial: increase time to 10–30 min q 3 h	Same as Day 2 except • Wt • Weaning trial: increase time to 30–60 min q 3 h	Same as Day 3 Weaning trial: increase time 2–3 h QID W/A	Same as Day 4 except: Wt Weaning trial: increase time to 3–4 h off, followed by 1–2 h on	Same as Day 5 Weaning trial: increase time to 4–6 h off and 1–2 h on	I & O TCDB Pulmonary hygiene Exercise program to increase strength and endurance

Nutrition	Nutritional assessment Calorie count x 3 day Possible need for supplement PO: high protein, high fat, low carbohydrate TPN or enteral feeding if unable to take PO feeding Increase fluids unless contra-indicated	Same as Day 1	Same as Day 2	Same as Day 3	Same as Day 4	Same as Day 5	Begin DAT
Lines/Tubes/ Monitors	IV for TPN IV saline loc NGT or gastros-tomy if unable to take PO fluids	Same as Day 1	Same as Day 2	Same as Day 3	Same as Day 4	Same as Day 5	Convert to saline loc
Mobility/ Self-Care	Up in chair BID	Up in chair TID	Up in chair to hall or patient lounge	Same as Day 3	Same as Day 4	Ambulate in room	Ambulate in hall
Discharge Planning	Social worker to assess need for social services, financial status, health insurance and coverage, home environ-ment, need for placement and family support	Evaluate insur-ance coverage for home health, sub-acute care, NH/rehab facility	Continue as Day 1 and 2	Same as Day 3	Same as Day 4	Same as Day 5	Ensure needed equipment ready and home modifications made, if needed Prepare paper work for transfer, if needed

Appendix

A

Patient Pathways

▼ ▼ ▼

Patient Pathway for Asthma

NOTE: This is a guideline for care only. Your care will be specific to meet your needs.

Aspect of Care	Date____ Day 1	Date____ Day 2	Date____ Day 3
Assessment	Your doctor or nurse will do a physical exam. Your nurse will listen to your lungs and heart at the start of each shift. Your vital signs (blood pressure, temperature, pulse and breathing) will be checked every 4 hours. You will be given a container to place your sputum/spit into. Your sputum will be checked for color and how much there is. We will check you frequently to be sure you are not having more trouble breathing.	Your doctor or nurse will do a physical exam. Your nurse will listen to your lungs and heart at the start of each shift. Your vital signs (blood pressure, temperature, pulse, and breathing) will be checked every 4 hours. You will be given a container to place your sputum/spit into. Your sputum will be checked for color and how much there is. We will check you frequently to be sure you are not having more trouble breathing.	Your doctor or nurse will do a physical exam. Your nurse will listen to your lungs and heart at the start of each shift. Your vital signs (blood pressure, temperature, pulse and breathing) will be checked every 8 hours. You will be given a container to place your sputum/spit into. Your sputum will be checked for color and how much there is. We will check you frequently to be sure you are not having more trouble breathing.
Teaching	You and your family will be prepared for all tests and procedures. You will be told: · Name of test · Why it is being done · Where and when it will be done · Who will do it · What you should do during the test · What the test is like (discomfort, noises, etc.) We will provide you with information about your diagnosis.	You will be taught how to reduce stress and exercises to do when you feel stressed. We will teach you or review with you how to recognize and prevent infections. We will teach you several things you can do when you are having trouble breathing to make breathing easier.	You will be given information concerning diet, exercise, and medication you will take when you go home. We will give you a booklet that talks about things that might trigger an asthma attack and what you can do to prevent an attack.

	Day 1		
	We will tell you how we plan to care for you and ask you to tell us how you would like to be cared for. You will receive information on how to use an inhaler and nebulizer which are used to give you medication to make breathing easier.		
Consults	Your doctor may ask a doctor who specializes in breathing problems to see you. A respiratory therapist will help you with your breathing treatments.	Same as Day 1.	None.
Lab Tests	Blood will be drawn from a vein in your arm. Blood will be drawn from an artery in your wrist. This may cause mild discomfort. Some of your sputum from a deep cough will be checked to see if you have an infection in your lungs.	Blood will be drawn from a vein in your arm.	Same as yesterday.
Other Tests	A chest x-ray will be done. An EKG will be done if you are over 40 years old. Tests called pulmonary function tests will be done to see how well your lungs are doing. These tests do not cause discomfort.	None.	None.

Continued

Patient Pathway for Asthma Continued

Aspect of Care (Cont'd)	Date____ Day 1	Date____ Day 2	Date____ Day 3
Medications	You will be given medication through your IV line. Other medications to help you breathe easier will be given to you with your breathing treatments. We will tell you the name of the medication, why you are getting it, and what it is for.	Your IV medications may be changed to a type you can take by mouth. You will continue to receive medication with your breathing treatments.	All medications will be taken by mouth.
Treatments	You may be given oxygen to help you breathe better. We will explain to you how this works. **You may not smoke or light a match when oxygen is used.** You will start nebulizer treatments to help you breathe better. They will be explained to you when they are done. They do not cause any discomfort. A small cap-like device called a pulse oximeter will be placed on your finger to help us know how much oxygen you are getting. This does not cause any discomfort, and you can move your hand without any trouble. It will be explained to you when put on. An IV (small needle placed in a vein in your arm) may be inserted to give you medications.	If you do not need it anymore, your oxygen will be stopped. The breathing treatments will continue. The device (pulse oximeter) on your finger may be stopped. The IV will be removed.	Your oxygen will be stopped. You will be taught how to use an inhaler at home to help you breathe easier. The pulse oximeter will be stopped.

	Your diet will be the same as it was at home unless you are on steroid medication. In that case your salt intake may be limited. Staff will discuss your diet with you to help you choose foods you like.		
Mobility	You may get up to go to the bathroom. You may sit on the side of the bed if it helps you breathe easier.	You may get up in the chair or walk around in your room or in the hallway.	You may walk around your room and in the hallway.
Discharge Planning	Staff will help you decide if you need to make any modifications in your home or daily schedule as a result of your asthma attack.	Same as yesterday.	Staff will assist you to make a follow-up appointment to see your doctor after you are home.

Patient Pathway for Uncomplicated Myocardial Infarction

NOTE: This is a guideline for care only. Your care will be specific to meet your needs.

Aspect of Care	Date____ Day 1	Date____ Day 2	Date____ Day 3	Date____ Day 4
Assessment	You will be admitted to the critical care unit and connected to a machine (heart monitor) that will let your doctor and nursing staff know how your heart is beating. The staff will observe you carefully and take your vital signs (like blood pressure) very frequently. The nurse or respiratory therapist will use a small device to attach to your finger or ear lobe to check the amount of oxygen in your blood. This will be done several times through the next few days.	Your close monitoring will continue today. Assessment is similar to yesterday.	You should be transferred to a "stepdown" unit or telemetry unit today. Your heart will continue to be monitored in these units. Your vital signs will be taken every 4–8 hours.	The nursing staff will take your vital signs every 8 hours and check you for chest pain. Your chest will be connected to a heart monitor until discharge from the hospital.
Teaching	The staff will explain to you what happened and explain all procedures and treatments (including this patient pathway). You should report any chest pains or other unusual sensations to a nurse immediately.	Your nurse or nurse specialist will begin teaching you more about what a myocardial infarction (heart attack) is and the need to conserve your energy and limit activity.	Cardiac teaching will continue today, including information about diet, medications, and the need to monitor daily weight. Report chest pain or other unusual sensations. Be sure to ask questions and voice any concerns.	The nurse and other staff will review discharge instructions regarding: • Chest pain episodes • Medications • Diet • Physical activity allowance and progression

You may feel a little confused because your heart cannot pump enough blood to your brain.	Report chest pain or other unusual sensations. Be sure to ask questions and voice any concerns.		• Sexual activity • Reduction of risk factors (such as smoking, weight loss)
Consults A heart specialist (cardiologist) may be asked to see you. A cardiac rehabilitation nurse may visit you today or tomorrow.	A social worker may visit you to discuss your home situation, financial needs, or discharge plans.	A dietician may see you to discuss special dietary needs.	None.
Lab Tests Your blood will be drawn frequently to check for chemical levels, "low" blood, and enzymes that indicate how your heart is working. A urine sample may also be requested.	Your blood will be drawn today for testing.	Your blood will be drawn today for testing.	None.
Other Tests You will have a chest x-ray and several electrocardiograms (ECG), which show the electrical activity of your heart.	You may have other tests on Day 1 or 2 to check your heart, such as an echocardiogram (sonogram that uses sound waves).	Your doctor may order a cardiac catheterization. This test is done in a special lab to allow your doctor to see specific blockages in your heart.	You may have an ECG or special ECG while you walk on a treadmill (stress test). This test may be scheduled for a later date.
Meds If you are a candidate, your doctor or Emergency Room doctor may give you an IV drug to dissolve the clot that is causing your MI. You will receive a strong pain killer (morphine) to relieve your chest pain and help your heart.	You may receive an anti-coagulant ("blood thinner"). The nursing staff will observe you carefully for bleeding. Your other heart drugs will continue, but doses may be changed depending on your need.	Continue with heart medications (most or all will be by pill form by today). Continue with stool softener.	You will continue your current medications.

Continued

Patient Pathway for Uncomplicated Myocardial Infarction *Continued*

Aspect of Care (Cont'd)	Date ___ Day 1	Date ___ Day 2	Date ___ Day 3	Date ___ Day 4
Meds (Cont'd)	You will also receive many heart medications—some in pill form, some in IV form, and some may be put on your skin.	You will receive a stool softener to prevent straining during a bowel movement.		
Treatments	You will receive some oxygen through small nasal prongs/tubing. Your fluid intake and urine output will be measured. You will probably be weighed every day. You will receive continuous IV fluids. You should be able to eat and drink. Your doctor and dietitian will most likely prescribe a special low salt and/or low fat diet.	Same as yesterday.	Today your IV fluids will be discontinued, but the needle will be capped for use as needed later. The staff will no longer measure your intake and output. Continue on cardiac monitoring.	Care is the same as Day 3 until you leave the hospital.
Mobility/Self-Care	You will probably be allowed out of bed with assistance to use a bedside commode. The staff will help you with bathing or other activities as you need them.	Your doctor will probably allow you up in a chair for 30 minutes 2–3 times a day, per cardiac rehabilitation protocol.	You should be up to ambulating in your room and using the bathroom.	You should walk in the hall, but don't overtire yourself. Allow rest periods as needed.

Discharge Planning			
The staff will begin assessing your home situation for special needs and support after hospital discharge. You and your family will be an active part in discharge planning.	If needed, a social worker/nurse will begin making arrangements for home health services, such as homemaking, nursing, and physical therapy. If a rehabilitation or long-term care facility is necessary, the discharge planners will make the necessary arrangements with the help of family or other caregivers.	Continue with Day 2.	A follow-up appointment with your doctor will be made. Arrangements for lab tests and further heart tests will also be made for you for follow-up evaluation.

Patient Pathway for Cerebral Vascular Accident

NOTE: This is a guideline for care only. Your care will be specific to meet your needs.

Aspect of Care	Date____ Day 1	Date____ Day 2	Date____ Day 3	Date____ Day 4
Assessment	Your doctor and nurse will do a physical exam. Your nurse will do a brief physical exam at the start of each shift. Your vital signs (blood pressure, pulse, temperature, and respirations) will be checked every 1–2 hours for the first day. Your neuro signs will be checked every 1–2 hours. This means we will: • Ask you to move your arms and legs and see how strong they are • Shine a light in your eyes to see how they react • Check your vision • Ask you several questions We will check you frequently to prevent or treat possible complications.	Your doctor and nurse will do a brief physical exam each day. Your vital signs will be taken every 4 hours. Your neuro signs will be checked every 4 hours. We will check you frequently to prevent or treat possible complications.	Your doctor and nurse will do a brief physical exam. Your vital signs will be taken every 4 hours. Your neuro signs will be checked every 4 hours. We will check you frequently to prevent or treat possible complications.	Vital signs will be checked in the morning and evening. The nurse will do a brief physical examination.

Teaching	The staff will tell you about the hospital and visiting policies. You and your family will be prepared for all tests and procedures. You and the family will be told: • The name of the test • Why it is being done • Where and when it will be done • Who will do it • What you should do during the test • What the test is like (loud noises, discomfort) We will provide you and your family with information about your diagnosis. We will tell you how we plan to care for you and will ask you and your family what we can do to make your stay with us more comfortable.	We will continue to teach you about your diagnosis and to prepare you for tests. Please continue to let us know what we can do to make your stay better for you and your family.	We will help you learn to adapt to any problems you may have taking care of yourself. We will teach you things you can do to take care of yourself and prevent another stroke by changing your diet, exercising, and stopping smoking if you are a smoker.	We will review your exercise program and plans for discharge home or to a rehabilitation center.
Consults	Your doctor may ask other doctors and therapists to see you.	The physical therapist will visit you today to help you learn how to strengthen the muscles that are weak. The occupational therapist will visit you to see if you need equipment to help you to care for yourself.	The physical therapist, occupational therapist, and speech therapist will continue to visit you and give you therapy.	None.

Continued

Patient Pathway for Cerebral Vascular Accident *Continued*

Aspect of Care (Cont'd)	Date_____ Day 1	Date_____ Day 2	Date_____ Day 3	Date_____ Day 4
Consults (Cont'd)		The speech therapist will visit you if you have trouble swallowing or speaking. The dietician will help you learn more about diet and the kinds of foods you should have in your diet.		
Lab Tests	Blood will be taken from a vein in your arm. The nurse will tell you what these tests are for.	Blood will be taken from a vein in your arm.	Blood will be taken from a vein in your arm.	None.
Other Tests	You will have a CT scan or MRI scan, which are specialized x-rays of your head. They are not uncomfortable and do not cause pain. Your doctor and nurse will explain the tests to you, and the technician doing the test will give you more information as the test is done. A chest x-ray will be done. An ECG will be done.	You may have a Doppler or ultrasonic test today to see how well blood flows to your head. These tests are not painful. An EEG may be done today as well as an echocardiogram. These tests are not painful. The staff will explain these tests to you before they occur.	No special test will be done today.	None.

Meds	Medications may be given to you through your IV line. You may be given other medications to take by mouth if you do not have trouble swallowing. We will tell you the name of all medications and why you are getting them.	You will continue to get medications. You will get more information about the medications you are taking.	You will continue to receive medications. You will get more information about the medications you are taking.	You will be given information about the medications you will take at discharge.
Treatments	An intravenous line (IV) will be inserted into a vein in your arm to give you fluids and medications. Special stockings called TEDS will be placed on your legs. Your nurse will explain their purpose when they are put on. You will be helped to turn and asked to take deep breaths every 2 hours. You will not be given anything to eat or drink until we are sure you do not have any trouble swallowing. If you have trouble swallowing, an x-ray will be done on Day 2 or 3 to find out where the problem is.	The IV will remain in place although you may not receive any fluids in it. Stockings will be removed twice each day for 1 hour. Salt may be restricted in your diet. You will be given foods that you can swallow. We will continue to measure your fluids or I & O.	Your IV will remain in place although you may not receive any fluids in it. Stockings will be removed twice each day for 1 hour. We will continue to give you foods that are easy for you to chew and swallow. The dietician will give you and your family information about the diet that is best for you and what foods you may make at home to stay on this diet. We will continue to measure your I & O.	We will continue the same treatments as yesterday.

Continued

Patient Pathway for Cerebral Vascular Accident *Continued*

Aspect of Care (Cont'd)	Date ___ Day 1	Date ___ Day 2	Date ___ Day 3	Date ___ Day 4
Treatments (Cont'd)	We will measure how much fluid you drink and how much urine you make. We call this measuring your intake and output, or I & O.			
Mobility/Self-Care	You must remain in bed today. The staff will assist you to use the bathroom. You will be assisted to move your arms and legs to prevent your muscles from getting stiff and sore. The head of your bed will be raised slightly. We will help you turn and get into a comfortable position.	You will be assisted to the chair and to use the bathroom. We will show you and your family how to move the arm and leg that is weak and exercises to improve strength.	You will be assisted to the chair and to use the bathroom. We will continue to show you how to increase the strength of the weak arm and leg. The therapist will assist you with walking in your room or in the therapy room.	You may get up in the chair four times a day or more often if you want to. The therapist will continue to help you with rehabilitation.
Discharge Planning	A social worker will see you to discuss any concerns you may have.	The staff will help you decide on where you should go after discharge. This may be home or to a rehabilitation facility. We will tell you about rehabilitation and help you and your family find a place that is best for you.	If you are going home, we will assist your family to obtain needed equipment or to make modifications to your home. If you are going to a rehabilitation facility, we will send them all the information they need to take care of you and get your rehabilitation program moving along.	We will make sure all arrangements for your discharge are done. We will arrange for any follow-up visits with your doctor.

Notes

Patient Pathway for Total Hip Replacement

NOTE: This is a guideline for care only. Your care will be specific to meet your needs.

Aspect of Care	Date____ Pre-admission/ Pre-op	Date____ Day 1	Date____ Day 2	Date____ Day 3	Date____ Day 4	Date____ Day 5-6
Assessment	Before surgery, a nurse in the operating room will review the procedure with you. You will have a brief physical exam to check that everything is OK before surgery. The nurse will ask you some questions and take your vital signs (temperature, pulse, respirations, and blood pressure). You will also be asked to sign a paper giving permission to do the surgery.	When surgery is over, you will wake up in the Recovery Room (now called the Post-Anesthesia Care Unit or PACU). The nurses in PACU will check your vital signs about every 15 minutes at first. You will be awakened and checked very frequently. When you are fully awake, you will be transferred to a hospital unit. There you can have medication for pain and you will continue to be checked carefully every 30–60 minutes.	A nurse or other staff member will check your vital signs and hip dressing, listen to your chest, and listen for bowel sounds at least every 8 hours. You will also be monitored for the amount of fluid you drink or receive in your IV. Your urine will also be measured. The nurse will check your skin, especially your heels, and make sure that you follow the recommended hip precautions (avoid crossing legs, turn only to unaffected side using pillow between legs).	The nursing staff will continue to check your vital signs, breath sounds, bowel sounds, skin, legs, and incision several times each day. You will be asked whether or not you have had a bowel movement.	The staff will continue to check you frequently as they have done each day.	The staff will continue to check you frequently.

Teaching	Your doctor and office staff will teach you what a total hip replacement is and what you can expect after surgery. Things you can expect after surgery will also be discussed, such as pain management, activity, hip precautions, medications, and IVs. This entire pathway should be reviewed with you and your family. A physical therapist may also teach you how to use a walker and exercises that you will do after surgery.	You will be reminded to do deep breathing and coughing at least every 2 hours. You will also need to use the incentive spirometer every 2 hours. Someone will show you how to use it. Your nurse will teach you about pain management techniques, anticoagulant drug therapy (blood "thinner"), hip precautions, and leg exercises (ankle pumps, quad and gluteal sets). You might feel a little confused for the rest of today as the anesthesia wears off.	Feel free to ask any questions or voice any concerns that you have. The nurse will review the information that was previously taught.	The nurse will begin discussing discharge plans and the care that will be needed if you are going home.	The nurse and physical therapist will begin discharge teaching regarding: • Incision care • Pain management • Physical activity/sexual activity • Ambulation/weight-bearing • Exercises • Rehabilitation program • Medications • Hip precautions • Bleeding precautions/testing
				The nurse will review the discharge instructions and answer any questions you have.	
Consults	A physical therapist and possibly an occupational therapist may evaluate you for special needs that you will have after surgery, such as a platform walker instead of a standard walker.	A social worker may evaluate you for the need to have inpatient or outpatient rehabilitation after discharge from the hospital.	A physical therapist will visit you to review the leg exercises that you need to do and determine your progress since surgery.	A physical therapist will begin working with you on weight-bearing, gait training, and ambulation.	None.
					None.

Continued

Patient Pathway for Total Hip Replacement *Continued*

Aspect of Care (Cont'd)	Date ___ Pre-admission/Pre-op	Date ___ Day 1	Date ___ Day 2	Date ___ Day 3	Date ___ Day 4	Date ___ Day 5–6
Lab Tests	You will need to come to the lab several days before surgery to have blood drawn to make sure you don't have "low" blood (anemia) and that you do not bleed easily.	Your blood will be drawn in the evening for testing.	Your blood will be drawn this morning.	Your blood will be drawn today.	Your blood will be drawn today.	Your blood will be drawn.
Other Tests	You'll be asked to have a chest x-ray and electro-cardiogram (heart test).	Your doctor may order an x-ray of your hip while you are in the PACU.	None.	Your doctor may order a hip x-ray today.	None.	None.
Meds	Before surgery you will have an IV to provide fluids and a way to give medications, such as an antibiotic to prevent infection and drugs to make you sleepy before you receive anesthesia.	After surgery, your doctor will order more antibiotic doses (2–4) and pain medication.	You will still receive pain medication. You will also probably start your blood thinner today to prevent blood clots. You can have a stool softener at bedtime.	If you have not had a bowel movement by today, you will receive a laxative. You can have pain pills or an injection if needed. You will continue on your blood thinner. If needed, you can have a stool softener.	You can have pain pills when you need them. Your therapy will continue. If needed, you can have a stool softener.	Medications same as yesterday.

Treatments				
You will be asked to scrub your thigh and hip with Betadine the night before surgery. You will also not be allowed to eat or drink anything or to smoke from 12 midnight the night before surgery. If you have been taking aspirin, ibuprofen, or similar drug, you will be asked to stop taking them for several days prior to surgery. Immediately before surgery, you will have an IV inserted. Your doctor may also order a Foley urinary catheter during the surgery only.	After surgery, you will have a pillow or other device between your legs to prevent hip dislocation. You will be assisted to turn, cough, and deep breathe every 2 hours. You will also be reminded to use the incentive spirometer every 2 hours. Someone will record how much fluid you take in and how much urine you excrete. You will have thigh-high antiembolism stockings and sequential compression devices (SCDs) on both legs to prevent clots. These devices are a little noisy and warm. The nursing staff will assist you in moving your nonoperative leg and arms to prevent them from getting stiff.	Your care for today will be similar to yesterday's care. If you are not nauseated, you may have liquids today. You will keep your IV to provide continuous fluids so that you don't get dehydrated. The drain in your hip will be emptied and measured every 8 hours.	Your hip dressing will be changed and the drain will be removed by your doctor. You need to continue using hip precautions and wearing your antiembolism stockings. You can eat whatever you like unless you are on a special diet. Your IV will be removed today.	The nurse or technician will change your dressing or clean your incision several times a day. You can eat whatever you like unless you are on a special diet.	Care is the same as yesterday.

Continued

Patient Pathway for Total Hip Replacement Continued

Aspect of Care (Cont'd)	Date____ Pre-admission/ Pre-op	Date____ Day 1	Date____ Day 2	Date____ Day 3	Date____ Day 4	Date____ Day 5–6
Treatments (Cont'd)		If you cannot pass your water, you may have a catheter to empty your bladder. You cannot have anything to eat or drink until you are fully awake. Then you can have some clear liquids.				
Mobility/Self-Care	You may have activity as tolerated.	You will stay in bed today in a reclining position. If you need to toilet, a special small bedpan will be used to make movement more comfortable. You will have a frame and trapeze on your bed so that you can help to move yourself. You will need to do exercises for your legs as taught.	Today you will be assisted to sit on the side of the bed. Then you will be helped from the bed to a chair. Your operative leg will be elevated while you are out of bed. Hip precautions, such as not crossing your legs or feet and avoiding bending forward, will be reviewed with you.	You can be up in a chair with assistance several times today. You will go to the physical therapy (PT) department several times today for exercises to begin gait training and ambulation with a walker. You should use a bedside commode or a toilet with an elevated seat.	You can be up in your room using a walker bearing only a little weight on your operative leg (PT will show you how much weight to bear). You go to the PT department twice today for continued training using the walker.	Same as yesterday.

Discharge Planning					
None.	The social worker and nurse will talk with you about your care after discharge. Depending on your overall condition and home situation, you may go home, or to a rehabilitation center/unit for 4–6 weeks.	Continue with Day 1.	A social worker and nurse, working with the doctor, will discuss discharge plans with you. They will make arrangements for transfer to a rehabilitation facility or home.	If you go home, you will be seen by a nurse and physical therapist several times a week. Depending on your situation, you will visit a PT as an outpatient when able.	A follow-up appointment will be made for you with your doctor. The hospital staff will communicate your needs and care to the care providers who will see you after discharge from the hospital.

Patient Pathway for Acute Renal Failure: Peritoneal Dialysis

NOTE: This is a guideline for care only. Your care will be specific to meet your needs.

Aspect of Care	Date ___ Day 1	Date ___ Day 2	Date ___ Day 3	Date ___ Day 4	Date ___ Day 5
Assessment	Your doctor and nurse will do a physical exam. Your nurse will do a brief physical exam at the start of each shift. Your vital signs (blood pressure, temperature, pulse and breathing rate) will be checked every 4 hours and more frequently while you are receiving dialysis treatment. Your neurologic signs will be checked every 4 hours. This means we will: • Ask you to move your arms and legs to check how strong they are • Shine a light in your eyes to see how they react • Ask you several questions	Your doctor and nurse will do a physical exam. Your nurse will do a brief physical exam at the start of each shift. Your vital signs will be checked every 4 hours. Your neurologic signs will be checked every 4 hours. We will check you frequently to make sure there are no problems with the dialysis procedure such as the catheter being kinked or the dressing getting wet. Your doctor will continue to adjust your medication to get the dose that is best for you.	Care is the same as yesterday.	Care is the same as Day 2.	Care is the same as Day 2.

Teaching			
We will check you frequently to make sure there are no problems with the dialysis procedure such as discomfort, the catheter being kinked, or the dressing getting wet. Your doctor will adjust your medications to make sure you get the dose that is best for you. You and your family will be prepared for the peritoneal dialysis procedures. You will be told: • Why it is being done • How the peritoneal (abdominal) catheter will be inserted • How and when dialysis will be done • Who will do it • What you should do during dialysis • What dialysis feels like	The staff will continue to provide you with information about your diagnosis, peritoneal dialysis, and treatment plan.	You will receive information concerning your diet, rest, and exercise. Information will be provided concerning the medications you will need to take at discharge. You will be told: • Name of medications • How and when to take them • What they are for • What the possible side effects may be and what to do should they occur	We will review all information you need for discharge. Your diet and medications will be reviewed with you. The staff will teach you and your family how to do peritoneal dialysis at home if necessary: • How to perform • What to do and who to call for problems • How to care for equipment • How to prevent infection You will receive a booklet explaining diet, medication, exercise and activity, and rest.

Continued

Patient Pathway for Acute Renal Failure: Peritoneal Dialysis *Continued*

Aspect of Care (Cont'd)	Date ___ Day 1	Date ___ Day 2	Date ___ Day 3	Date ___ Day 4	Date ___ Day 5
Teaching (Cont'd)	We will tell you how we plan to care for you and ask you to tell us what we can do to help you feel better. You will be given information concerning your diagnosis.				
Consults	Your physician may ask other doctors to see you, for example, a doctor who specializes in kidney disease (nephrologist).	The dietician will see you to discuss your diet. Our social worker will help you with understanding insurance and financial issues and can help you arrange care at home.	Same as yesterday.	None.	None.
Lab Tests	Blood will be drawn from a vein in your arm on admission to the hospital and after each dialysis procedure. A urine sample (if applicable) will be sent to check for infection. Fluid from the catheter in your abdomen will be checked for infection.	Blood will be drawn from a vein in your arm.	Blood will be drawn from a vein in your arm.	Blood will be drawn from a vein in your arm. Fluid from the catheter in your abdomen will be checked for infection.	Blood will be drawn from a vein in your arm.

Other Tests	An x-ray of your chest and kidneys will be taken. A special x-ray called a CT scan or MRI may be done. An ECG will be done. None of these tests will cause you any discomfort.	No tests today.	No tests today.	None.	None.
Meds	You will be given a vitamin with iron. Your doctor will order other medication, and we will tell you what it is for and how often you are to get it.	Medications same as yesterday.	Medications same as Day 1.	Medications same as on Day 1.	Medications same as on Day 1.
Treatments	Before peritoneal dialysis: • Your vital signs will be taken • The nurse will measure the size of your abdomen/waist • You will be asked to try to urinate • You will be weighed During dialysis • Your vital signs will be taken	You will receive the same care before, during, and after dialysis as yesterday. We will continue to measure your I & O. Your diet may be changed a little depending on your response to dialysis.	Same as yesterday. Your diet will be adjusted to meet your individual needs.	Treatment same as Day 1.	Same as on Day 1 if still require dialysis. IV will be discontinued.

Continued

Patient Pathway for Acute Renal Failure: Peritoneal Dialysis *Continued*

Aspect of Care (Cont'd)	Date ___ Day 1	Date ___ Day 2	Date ___ Day 3	Date ___ Day 4	Date ___ Day 5
Treatments (Cont'd)	• We will be sure that the tubing is not kinked or obstructed in any way • If you have any discomfort or trouble breathing, tell the nurse After dialysis: • Your vital signs will be taken • Blood will be drawn from a vein in your arm • Your abdomen will be measured You will be placed on I & O, which means that we measure all the liquids you drink as well as things such as Jello, ice chips, ice cream that are liquids at room temperature. We will measure the amount of urine each time you go to the bathroom. The dietician will discuss your diet with you and help you to select foods low in salt and postassium and includes the right amount of protein for you.				

	The amount of fluid you can drink will be limited. The staff will help you to select when and what you would like to drink. An IV needle will be placed in a vein in your arm.				
Mobility/Self-Care	You may be out of bed to use the bathroom.	You may sit up in a chair as long as you are comfortable.	You may be out of bed and walk in the halls as you feel up to it.	Activity same as Day 3.	Activity same as Day 3.
Discharge Planning	Staff will talk to you about insurance and other financial considerations.	Staff will assist you and your family to make necessary arrangements for things you may need at discharge.	Same as yesterday.	We will continue to help you and your family identify any changes needed.	Same as yesterday.

Patient Pathway for Total Abdominal Hysterectomy

NOTE: This is a guideline for care only. Your care will be specific to meet your needs.

Aspect of Care	Date_____ Pre-admission/Pre-op	Date_____ Day 1	Date_____ Day 2	Date_____ Day 3
Assessment	Before surgery, a nurse in the operating room will review the procedure with you. You will have a brief physical exam to check that everything is OK before surgery. The nurse will ask you some questions and take your temperature, respirations, pulse, and blood pressure. You will also be asked to sign a paper giving permission to do the surgery.	When surgery is over, you will wake up in the Recovery Room (now called the Post-Anesthesia Care Unit, or PACU). The nurses in PACU will check your vital signs (blood pressure, pulse) about every 15 minutes at first. You will be awakened and checked very frequently. When you are fully awake, you will be transferred to a hospital unit. There you can have medication for pain and you will continue to be checked carefully every 30–60 minutes.	A nurse will check your vital signs and abdominal surgical dressing, listen to your chest, and listen for bowel sounds at least every 8 hours. You will also be monitored for the amount of fluid you drink or receive in your IV. Your urine will be measured until you urinate without difficulty. Your perineal pad (sanitary napkin) will be checked frequently for bleeding.	The nursing staff will continue to check your abdomen, chest, and vital signs. You will also be asked to let the staff know when you have a bowel movement.
Teaching	Your doctor and office staff will teach you about what a hysterectomy is and what you can expect after surgery. Things you can expect after surgery will also be discussed, such as pain	You will be reminded to do deep breathing and coughing at least every 2 hours. You will also need to use the incentive spirometer every 2 hours and someone will show you how to use it.	You may be taught some additional pain relief measures, such as muscle relaxation and visual imagery. These techniques do not take the place of pain medication but might decrease the amount of medicine needed.	The nurse will review information that you will need before you go home. Be sure to ask any questions that you have.

Consults	management, care of your incision, IVs, and Foley catheter. This entire pathway should be reviewed with you and your family.	Report any unusual sensations or bleeding to your nurse or aide/technician. Feel free to ask questions or voice any concerns that you might have.	None.	The nurse will begin to review discharge instructions about wound care, pain management activity, physical changes, and medications at home.
Lab Tests	You will need to come to the lab several days before surgery to have blood drawn to make sure you do not have "low" blood (anemia) and that you do not bleed easily.	A lab technician will draw your blood this evening or early in the morning to check for anemia.	None.	None.
Other Tests	You will be asked to have a chest x-ray and electrocardiogram (heart test) if you are over 40 or have a heart problem.	None.	None.	None.
Meds	Before surgery you will have an IV to provide fluids and a way to give medications, such as an antibiotic to prevent infection and drugs to make you sleepy before you receive anesthesia.	After surgery, your doctor will order pain medication to be given by injection (a needle) or in your IV by a patient-controlled analgesia (PCA) pump. A nurse will show you how to use this machine so that you can give yourself pain medication when needed. You may also receive more IV antibiotics and can have medication for nausea if this occurs.	If you had a PCA pump, it will probably be removed today. You still can have pain medication in pill form.	If you have not had a bowel movement by today, you will probably have a suppository or enema to make sure that your bowels are working.

Continued

Patient Pathway for Total Abdominal Hysterectomy *Continued*

Aspect of Care (Cont'd)	Date _____ Pre-admission/Pre-op	Date _____ Day 1	Date _____ Day 2	Date _____ Day 3
Treatments	Your physician or office staff should talk with you about how you feel regarding the surgery. You will be asked to avoid food, liquids, and smoking from 12 midnight the night before surgery. An IV will be started before surgery and a Foley catheter to drain your urine will be inserted.	You can expect the nursing staff to provide perineal care (cleaning your "private" area) at least every 8 hours. If your surgical abdominal dressing gets wet or loose, the staff will put a clean bandage over it for protection. Your urine bag will be emptied every 8 hours and the urine will be measured and recorded. Someone will help you change position, cough, and deep breathe about every 2 hours; you will need to use the incentive spirometer, too. After surgery you may be allowed to have a few ice chips or sips of water. Otherwise, you can not have anything to eat or drink because you will become nauseated and probably very sick.	You will be helped as needed with perineal care. You will need to continue changing positions, taking deep breaths, and using the spirometer. If you pass gas or have bowel sounds, you will be allowed to begin to eat food that you can tolerate. When you are eating and drinking without any problems, your IV will be taken out. Your urinary catheter will also be removed, and the staff will be checking to make sure that you void ("pass your water") without problem. You will be allowed to have clear liquids, like water, apple juice, and broth. By dinner time you can progress to full liquids, or any liquid that you like.	Your doctor will change or remove your surgical dressing today. You can eat or drink anything that you want.

Mobility/Self-Care	You will not have any restrictions on your activity before surgery.	If your surgery was early in the morning, you will probably be assisted out of bed into a chair sometime in the evening. You will be shown how to do leg exercises, including ankle pumps, to prevent a blood clot. You will have elastic stockings on to also help prevent blood clots.	You can be up in your room and to the bathroom today. If you need assistance or feel dizzy, call the staff for help. Your doctor may let you shower, but you should not get your surgical dressing wet.	You should get up and walk around today in your room and in the hall. This movement helps to decrease "gas pains." Your doctor may allow you to shower, but you need to keep your incision dry.
Discharge Planning	None.	A social worker or other discharge planner may talk with you about special needs and support that you will need at home.	Continue with Day 1.	Your doctor will give you a prescription for pain pills. You will also have an appointment to get your stitches or staples taken out.

Appendix
B

NANDA-Approved Nursing Diagnoses

▼ ▼ ▼

This list represents the nursing diagnoses approved by NANDA for clinical use and testing (1994).

Activity Intolerance
* Activity Intolerance, Risk for
# Adaptive Capacity: Intracranial, Decreased
Adjustment, Impaired
Airway Clearance, Ineffective
Anxiety
* Aspiration, Risk for
Body Image Disturbance
* Body Temperature, Risk for Altered
Breastfeeding, Effective
Breastfeeding, Ineffective
Breastfeeding, Interrupted
Breathing Pattern, Ineffective
Caregiver Role Strain
* Caregiver Role Strain, Risk for
Communication, Impaired Verbal
Community Coping, Ineffective
Community Coping, Potential for Enhanced
Confusion, Acute
Confusion, Chronic
Constipation
Constipation, Colonic
Constipation, Perceived
Decisional Conflict (Specify)
Decreased Cardiac Output
Defensive Coping
Denial, Ineffective
Diarrhea
Disorganized Infant Behavior
Disorganized Infant Behavior, Risk for
Disuse Syndrome, Risk for
Diversional Activity Deficit
Dysfunctional Ventilatory Weaning Response (DVWR)
Dysreflexia
Energy Field Disturbance
Environmental Interpretation Syndrome, Impaired
Family Coping: Compromised, Ineffective
Family Coping: Disabling, Ineffective
Family Coping: Potential for Growth
Family Processes: Alchoholism, Altered
Family Processes, Altered
Fatigue
Fear
Fluid Volume Deficit

* Fluid Volume Deficit, Risk for
Fluid Volume Excess
Gas Exchange, Impaired
Grieving, Anticipatory
Grieving, Dysfunctional
Growth and Development, Altered
Health Maintenance, Altered
Health Seeking Behaviors (Specify)
Home Maintenance Managment, Impaired
Hopelessness
Hyperthermia
Hypothermia
Incontinence, Bowel
Incontinence, Functional
Incontinence, Reflex
Incontinence, Stress
Incontinence, Total
Incontinence, Urge
Individual Coping, Ineffective
Infant Feeding Pattern, Ineffective
* Infection, Risk for
* Injury, Risk for
Knowledge Deficit (Specify)
Loneliness, Risk for
Management of Therapeutic Regimen: Community, Ineffective
Management of Therapeutic Regimen: Families, Ineffective
Management of Therapeutic Regimen: Individual, Effective
Management of Therapeutic Regimen (Individuals), Ineffective
Memory, Impaired
Noncompliance (Specify)
Nutrition: Less than Body Requirements, Altered
Nutrition: More than Body Requirements, Altered
Nutrition: Potential for More than Body Requirements, Altered
Oral Mucous Membrane, Altered
Organized Infant Behavior, Potential for Enhanced
Pain
Pain, Chronic
Parental Role Conflict
Parent/Infant/Child Attachment, Risk for Altered

#New diagnoses added in 1994 classified at level 1.4 using new Criteria for Staging.
*Diagnoses with modified label terminology in 1994. (This change was recommended by the NANDA Taxonomy Committee and adapted to remain consistent with the ICD.)
Copyright © 1995, North American Nursing Diagnosis Association.

Table continued on following page

325

Parenting, Altered
* Parenting, Risk for Altered
# Perioperative Positioning Injury, Risk for
* Peripheral Neurovascular Dysfunction, Risk for
Personal Identity Disturbance
Physical Mobility, Impaired
* Poisoning, Risk for
Post-Trauma Response
Powerlessness
Protection, Altered
Rape-Trauma Syndrome
Rape-Trauma Syndrome: Compound Reaction
Rape-Trauma Syndrome: Silent Reaction
Relocation Stress Syndrome
Role Performance, Altered
Self Care Deficit
  Bathing/Hygiene
  Dressing/Grooming
  Feeding
  Toileting
Self Esteem, Chronic Low
Self Esteem Disturbance
Self Esteem, Situational Low
* Self-Mutilation, Risk for
Sensory/Perceptual Alterations (Specify) (Visual, Auditory,

Kinesthetic, Gustatory, Tactile, Olfactory)
Sexual Dysfunction
Sexuality Patterns, Altered
Skin Integrity, Impaired
* Skin Integrity, Risk for Impaired
Sleep Pattern Disturbance
Social Interaction, Impaired
Social Isolation
Spiritual Distress (distress of the human spirit)
Spiritual Well-Being, Potential for Enhanced
* Suffocation, Risk for
Sustain Spontaneous Ventilation, Inability to
Swallowing, Impaired
Thermoregulation, Ineffective
Thought Processes, Altered
Tissue Integrity, Impaired
Tissue Perfusion, Altered (Specify Type) (Renal, Cerebral, Cardiopulmonary, Gastrointestinal, Peripheral)
* Trauma, Risk for
Unilateral Neglect
Urinary Elimination, Altered
Urinary Retention
* Violence: Self-Directed or Directed at Others, Risk for

Appendix
C

Spanish Patient Pathways

▼ ▼ ▼

Guía Para el Paciente: Asma

NOTA: Esta guía es solo para el cuidado general. Su cuidado será específico de acuerdo con sus necesidades.

Aspecto de Cuidado	Fecha_____ Día 1	Fecha_____ Día 2	Fecha_____ Día 3
Evaluación	El doctor o la(el) enfermera(o) le hará un examen físico.	El doctor o enfermera(o) le hará un examen físico.	El doctor o enfermera(o) le hará un examen físico.
	La(el) enfermera(o) escuchará los sonidos en los pulmones y en el corazón al inicio de cada turno.	La(el) enfermera(o) escuchará los sonidos en sus pulmones y en el corazón al inicio de cada turno.	La(el) enfermera(o) escuchará los sonidos en sus pulmones y en el corazón al inicio de cada turno.
	Se le tomarán los signos vitales (presión de sangre, pulso, temperatura, y respiración) cada cuatro (4) horas.	Se le tomarán los signos vitales (presión de sangre, temperatura, pulso y respiración) cada cuatro (4) horas.	Se le tomarán los signos vitales (presión de sangre, temperatura, pulso y respiración) cada ocho (8) horas.
	Se le dará un recipiente para que ponga la flema/escupa. Se observará la flema para notar la cantidad y el color.	Se le dará un recipiente para que ponga la flema/escupa. Se observará la flema para notar la cantidad y el color.	Se le dará un recipiente para que ponga la flema/escupa. Se observará la flema para notar la cantidad y el color.
	Le revisaremos con frecuencia para asegurarnos que no tiene más problemas al respirar.	Le revisaremos con frecuencia para asegurarnos que no tiene más problemas al respirar.	Le revisaremos con frecuencia para asegurarnos que no tiene más problemas al respirar.
Enseñanza (Instrucción)	Se le preparará a usted y a su familia para todas las pruebas de laboratorio y los procedimientos. Se le dará a conocer: • El nombre de la prueba • Porqué se hace • Cuándo y dónde se hace • Quién hace la prueba • Lo que usted debe hacer durante la prueba • Cómo es la prueba (ruidos, molestias, etc.)	Se le explicará como reducir la tensión y cómo hacer ejercicios cuando usted se sienta ansioso o con tensión. Le indicaremos o repasaremos con usted cómo reconocer las infecciones y cómo prevenirlas. Le recomendaremos varias cosas que usted puede hacer cuando tiente problemas al respirar. Esto mejorará la respiración.	Se le dará información acerca de la dieta (alimentos), ejercicios y medicinas que usted tomará cuando le den de alta. Le daremos un folleto que trata acerca de cosas que pueden causar o precipitar un ataque de asma y lo que usted puede hacer para prevenir un ataque.

	Le daremos información acerca de su diagnóstico.	
	Le diremos como planeamos su cuidado y le preguntaremos como quiere que le demos el cuidado.	
	Recibirá información de como usar un inhalador y nebulizador los cuales se usarán para darle la medicina que le ayudará a respirar mejor.	
Consultas	El doctor podrá llamar a un especialista en problemas respiratorios para que le revise a usted.	Igual que el día 1.	Ninguna.
	Un técnico en terapia respiratoria le ayudará con los tratamientos.	
Pruebas de Laboratorio	Le tomarán muestras de sangre de una vena del brazo.	Le tomarán muestras de sangre del brazo.	Igual que ayer.
	Le tomarán una muestra de sangre de una arteria en la muñeca del brazo. Esto le causará un poco de malestar.	
	Se examinará la flema que arroje cuando le digan que tosa fuerte para ver si tiene infección en los pulmónes.	
Otros Examenes	Le tomarán rayos-x del pecho.	Ninguno.	Ninguno.
	Le harán un electrocardiograma si es mayor de 40 años de edad.	
	Le harán pruebas de función pulmonar para ver cómo están trabajando los pulmónes. Estas pruebas no causan dolor o incapacitación.	

Guía Para el Paciente: Asma Continuada

Aspecto de Cuidado (Cont.)	Fecha_____ Día 1	Fecha_____ Día 2	Fecha_____ Día 3
Medicamentos	Le darán medicina por la vía intravenosa. Al mismo tiempo que le den el tratamiento respiratorio se le darán otras medicinas. Le diremos el nombre de la medicina, porque se le está administrando, y para qué es.	El medicamento por la vía intravenosa se cambiará por una medicina oral (que pueda tomar por la boca) Le continuarán dando su medicina junto con los tratamientos respiratorios.	Todos los medicamentos serán administrados por la boca (orales).
Tratamientos	Le darán oxígeno para que pueda respirar mejor. Le explicaremos cómo funciona. No podrá fumar o encender un cerillo/fósforo cuando use el oxígeno. Empezará a tomar tratamientos con el nebulizador para que respire mejor. Esto se le explicará antes de empezar. Los tratamientos no lo haran sentírse incómodo. Un aparatito que se llama oxímetro (pulse oximeter) se le pondrá en su dedo para que nos dé a saber cuánto oxígeno está circulando. Esto no causa malestar y usted podrá mover su mano sin problemas. Esto se le explicará al ponérselo. Una intravenosa (aguja chica que se introduce en una vena del brazo) se le colocará para darle medicamentos.	Si no necesita el oxígeno, se descontinuará. Se continuarán los tratamientos respiratorios. El oxímetro (pulse oximeter), se podrá descontinuar. La intravenosa se podrá descontinuar.	El oxígeno se descontinuará. Le mostrarán como usar el inhalador en casa para que le ayude a respirar mejor. Se descontinuará el oxímetro.

	Sus alimentos serán los mismos que toma cuando está en casa al menos que esté tomando esteroides. En ese caso, debe limitar la sal que toma. Las(os) enfermeras(os) le ayudarán a escojer los alimentos que le gusten.		
Movilidad/Auto Cuidado	Puede levantarse para ir al baño/sanitario. Puede sentarse al lado de la cama si esto le ayuda a respirar mejor.	Puede sentarse en la silla o caminar en su cuarto o en el pasillo.	Puede caminar en su cuarto o en el pasillo.
Plan al Darle de Alta	Ninguno.	Las(os) enfermeras(os) le ayudarán a decidir si necesita hacer cambios o modificaciones en su casa o en su horario diario debido al resultado del ataque de asma.	Las(os) enfermeras(os) le ayudarán a hacer una cita para que vea al doctor después que regrese a casa.

Guía Para el Paciente: Infarto al Miocardio sin Complicación

NOTA: Esta guía es solo para el cuidado general. Su cuidado será espcífico de acuerdo con sus necesidades.

Aspecto de Cuidado	Fecha_____ Día 1	Fecha_____ Día 2	Fecha_____ Día 3	Fecha_____ Día 4
Evaluación	Será admitido a la unidad de Terapia Intensiva y se le conectará a una máquina (monitor del corazón) que le indicará al doctor y a las(os) enfermeras(os) cómo está funcionando el corazón. Los empleados le observarán cuidadosamente y le tomarán los signos vitales (como la presión de sangre) con mucha frecuencia. La(el) enfermera(o) o el técnico de terapia respiratoria le pondrá un aparatito en su dedo o en la oreja para notar la cantidad de oxígeno en su sangre. Esto se hará varias veces al día por varios días.	Una evaluación estricta se continuará hoy. El examen físico es similar al de ayer.	Deberá ser trasladado hoy a una unidad de menos riesgo o de telemetría. Se le continuará el monitoreo del corazón en esas unidades. Se le tomarán los signos vitales cada cuatro a ocho (4–8) horas.	Los empleados de enfermería le tomarán los signos vitales cada ocho (8) horas y le haran preguntas acerca del dolor en el pecho. Le conectarán un monitor al pecho hasta que sea dado de alta del hospital.
Enseñanza (Instrucción)	Las(os) enfermeras(os) le comentarán que le sucedió y le explicarán todos los procedimientos y los tratamientos (incluyendo esta guía para el paciente).	La(el) enfermera(o) del piso o una especialista en enfermería clínica le empezará a dar instrucciones acerca de lo que es un infarto al miocardio (ataque al corazón) y la necesidad de conservar su energía y limitar las actividades.	El adiestramiento cardíaco (instrucciones) se empezará hoy, incluyendo información sobre los alimentos (dietas), medicamentos, y la necesidad de adquirir y anotar su peso diariamente.	La(el) enfermera(o) y otros empleados le darán instrucciones al ser dado de alta del hospital relacionadas con: • Episodios de dolor en el pecho • Medicamentos

	Deberá reportar cualquier dolor o sensaciones en el pecho a la(el) enfermera(o) inmediatamente. Es posible que se sienta un poco confuso ya que el corazón no está bombeando suficiente sangre hacia el cerebro.	Reporte cualquier dolor o sensaciones en el pecho. Por favor haga preguntas si tiene alguna duda.	Reporte el dolor o sensaciones raras en el pecho. Por favor haga preguntas si tiene alguna duda.	• Dieta (alimentos) • Actividad física (permitida y de progresión) • Actividad sexual • Reducción de factores de riesgo (tales como el fumar o la obesidad)
Consultas	Es posible que se le pida a un especialista en el corazón (cardiólogo) que le visite. Una enfermera en rehabilitación cardíaca le visitará hoy o mañana.	Un(una) trabajador(a) social le visitará para discutir su situación en casa, sus necesidades económicas o planes para cuando sea dado de alta del hospital.	Es posible que le visite una dietista para discutir sus alimentos o dietas especiales que necesite.	No se Aplica.
Pruebas de Laboratorio	Le tomarán muestras de sangre con frecuencia para notar niveles químicos, sangre "baja" (anemia), y las enzimas las cuales indican cómo está funcionando el corazón. También se le pedirá una muestra de orina.	Le tomarán muestras de sangre hoy para análisis.	Le tomarán muestras de sangre hoy para análisis.	No se Aplica.
Otros Examenes	Le tomarán rayos-x del pecho y varios electrocardiogramas (ECG) los cuales muestran la actividad del corazón.	Tal vez le tomen otras pruebas el primer o segundo día para examinar al corazón tales como un ecocardiograma (sonograma que usa ondas de sonido).	El doctor puede ordenar una prueba cardíaca. Esta prueba se hace en un laboratorio especial donde el doctor puede ver bloqueos específicos en el corazón.	Tal vez le tomen un electro-cardiograma o un electro-cardiograma especial mientras camina en una máquina (tread mill/prueba de esfuerzo). Esta prueba se planeará más tarde.

Continuada

Guía Para el Paciente: Infarto al Miocardio sin Complicación *Continuada*

Aspecto de Cuidado (Cont.)	Fecha_____ Día 1	Fecha_____ Día 2	Fecha_____ Día 3	Fecha_____ Día 4
Medicamentos	Se es candidato de poco riesgo; su doctor, o el doctor en el cuarto de emergencias, le dará un medicamento intravenoso para disolver el coágulo que le está causando el infarto. Recibirá una medicina fuerte para el dolor (Morfina) la cual le mejorará el dolor y le ayudará al corazón. También recibirá muchos medicamentos para el corazón; algunos en forma de pastilla, otros por vía intravenosa y otros que se deben aplicar a la piel.	Tal vez reciba anti-coagulantes (para adelgazar la sangre). Los empleados de enfermería observarán cuidadosamente si tiene hemorragias. Las otras medicinas para el corazón se descontinuarán, pero ciertas dósis tal vez se cambien de acuerdo con sus necesidades. Recibirá un laxante suave para prevenir el esfuerzo al obrar (al hacer del baño).	Continue tomando las medicinas para el corazón (la mayoria o todas serán en forma de pastilla/ pildoras). Continue tomando un laxante suave.	Continuará tomando las medicinas que le han recetado.
Tratamientos	Recibirá oxígeno por medio de puntas nasales/tubitos en la nariz. Se medirá la cantidad de líquidos que tome y la cantidad que orina. Se le tomará el peso todos los días. Se le aplicará un monitor cardíaco y recibirá fluidos intravenosos continuamente.	Igual que ayer.	Hoy los fluidos intravenosos se descontinuarán, pero la aguja se quedará para poder usarla más tarde. Los empleados de enfermería no tendrán que medir lo que tome o lo que orine. Continue con el monitor cardíaco.	Igual que el día 3 hasta que salga del hospital.

Movilidad/Auto Cuidado	Podrá tomar bebidas y comer. El doctor y la dietista le recetarán una dieta especial, baja en sal y/o baja en grasa.	Tal vez le permitan levantarse, con ayuda, para que use el sanitario/letrina al lado de la cama. Los empleados de enfermería le ayudarán a bañarse o a hacer otras actividades como sea necesario.	El doctor le permitirá sentarse en una silla por 30 minutos, dos o tres (2–3) veces por día, de acuerdo con el protocolo de rehabilitación cardíaca.	Podrá sentirse con fuerzas para caminar en su cuarto y usar el sanitario/letrina en el baño.	Deberá caminar en el pasillo, pero evite el cansancio. Descanse cuando sea necesario.
Plan al Darle de Alta		Los empleados de enfermería empezarán por evaluar la situación en su casa para apoyar sus necesidades después de ser dado de alta. Usted y su familia formarán parte integral del plan de cuidado.	Si es necesario, el(la) trabajador(a) social/la(el) enfermera(o) empezarán a hacer planes para prestarle servicios en casa (home health) tales como enfermería, ayuda con el quehacer y fisioterapia. Si es necesario trasladarle a un centro de cuidado crónico o de rehabilitación, las personas que planearán su salida del hospital harán los arreglos necesarios con ayuda de la familia o de otros profesionales.	Continue con el plan del día 2.	Se le harán citas con su doctor. Se harán arreglos para tomarle pruebas de laboratorio y otros exámenes del corazón para seguirle evaluando.	

Guía Para el Paciente: Remplazo Total de la Cadera

NOTA: Esta guía es solo para el cuidado general. Su cuidado será específico de acuerdo con sus necesidades.

Aspecto de Cuidado	Fecha ___ Pre-admisión/ Pre-operativo	Fecha ___ Día 1	Fecha ___ Día 2	Fecha ___ Día 3	Fecha ___ Día 4	Fecha ___ Día 5–6
Evaluación	Antes de la operación una(un) enfermera(o) en el quirófano repasará el procedimiento con usted. Le harán un examen físico breve para ver si todo está bien antes de la operación. La(el) enfermera(o) le dirá si tiene preguntas y le tomará los signos vitales (temperatura, pulso, respiración y la presión de sangre). Se le pedirá que firme una forma dando permiso para la operación.	Después de la operación, despertará en el cuarto/sala de recuperación (ahora se le llama unidad de post-anestesia o PACU). Las(os) enfermeras(os) en el PACU le tomarán los signos vitales cada 15 minutos al inicio de la estancia. Se le despertará y se evaluará su condición con mucha frecuencia. Cuando despierte por completo, se le transladará a un piso del hospital. Ahí podrá tomar medicina para el dolor y se le continuará evaluando cuidadosamente cada treinta a sesenta (30–60) minutos.	Una(un) enfermera(o) u otros empleados le tomarán los signos vitales, revisarán los bendajes en la cadera, y escucharán los sonido del pecho y de los intestinos al menos cada ocho (8) horas. También se anotará el volumen de líquidos que tome y lo que reciba en sueros intravenosos. La orina se medirá también. La(el) enfermera(o) observará la condición de la piel, especialmente de los talones y asegurará que usted siga las precauciones para la cadera (no cruce las piernas, volteese solo sobre el lado opuesto, coloque/póngase una almohada entre las piernas).	Las(os) enfermeras(os) le seguirán tomando varias veces cada día los signos vitales, escuchando los sonidos de la respiración y de los intestinos, y observando la piel y la incisión. Se le preguntará si ha obrado (hecho o no del baño).	Las(os) enfermeras(os) le seguirán revisando con frecuencia como lo hacen diariamente.	Las(os) enfermeras(os) le seguirán revisando con frecuencia.

Enseñanza (Instrucción)				
El doctor y los empleados de la oficina le darán instrucciones acerca del remplazo total de la cadera y lo que se espera desués de la operación. También discutirán lo que ocurrirá después de la operación, tal como el manejo del dolor, la movilidad, las precauciones para la cadera, los medicamentos y los sueros intravenosos. Esta guía para el paciente se deberá repasar con usted y con su familia. El técnico en fisioterapia trabajará con usted, especialmente para mostrarle como usar el andador y como hacer ejercicios.	Se le recordará que respire profundo y que tosa fuerte al menos cada dos (2) horas. También necesitará usar el inspiró-metro incentivo cada dos (2) horas y alguien le mostrará como usarlo. La enfermera le dará instrucciones sobre el manejo del dolor, los medicamentos anticoagulantes (adelgazamiento de la sangre), precauciones para la cadera, ejercicios para la pierna, el tobillo (punta y talón) y los músculos gluteales y sentadillas. Tal vez se sienta un poco confuso el resto del día hasta que se le pase la anestesia.	Por favor haga preguntas si tiene alguna duda o preocupación. La(el) enfermera(o) repasará con usted la información que se le dió antes de la operación.	La(el) enfermera(o) empezará a discutir con usted los planes para darle de alta y el cuidado que necesitará en casa.	La(el) enfermera(o) y el técnico de fisioterapia le darán instrucciones relacionadas con: • El cuidado de la herida (incisión) • El manejo del dolor • La actividad física/sexual • El caminar y poner peso • El ejercicio • El programa de rehabilitación • Los medica-mentos • Las precau-ciones para la cadera • Las precau-ciones contra hemorragias • Las pruebas o exámenes	La(el) enfermera(o) repasará con usted las instrucciones al darsele de alta y dará contestación a preguntas o dudas que tenga.

Continuada

Guía Para el Paciente: Remplazo Total de la Cadera *Continuada*

Aspecto de Cuidado (Cont.)	Fecha _____ Pre-admisión/ Pre-operativo	Fecha _____ Día 1	Fecha _____ Día 2	Fecha _____ Día 3	Fecha _____ Día 4	Fecha _____ Día 5-6
Consultas	Un(a) téchnico(a) en fisioterapia y tal vez un(a) terapeuta ocupacional lo evaluará para determinar si tendrá problemas especiales después de la operación, tales como el tipo de andador que necesitará.	Un(una) trabajador(a) social lo evaluará para ver si necesita rehabilitación en el hospital o en consulta externa después de ser dado de alta del hospital.	Un téchnico de fisioterapia le visitará para repasar con usted los ejercicios que necesita hacer y para determinar su progreso despues de la operación.	Un técnico en fisioterapia empezará a trabajar con usted y le mostrará la forma de andar, como poner peso, y como caminar.	Ninguna.	Ninguna.
Pruebas de Laboratorio	Tendrá que ir al laboratorio varios días antes de la operación para tomarle muestras de sangre. Esto indicará si tiene la sangre "baja" (anemia) y si se desangra fácilmente.	Le tomarán muestras de sangre por la tarde para hacerle análisis.	Le tomarán muestras de sangre esta mañana.	Le tomarán muestras de sangre hoy.	Le tomarán muestras de sangre hoy.	Le tomarán muestras de sangre.
Otros Examenes	Se le tomarán rayos-x del pecho y un electro-cardiograma (prueba del corazón).	Tal vez el doctor ordene que se le tomen rayos-x de la cadera mientras que esté en la unidad de post-anestesia (PACU).	No se Aplica.	El doctor tal vez ordene hoy rayos-x de la cadera.	Ninguno.	Ninguno.

Medicamentos	Antes de la operación le pondrán una intravenosa para administrarle fluidos y medicamentos tales como los antibióticos que previenen la infección y darle medicina que le adormecerá antes de recibir la anestesia.	Después de la operación, el doctor ordenará más dósis de antibióticos (2-4) y medicina para el dolor que puede darse usted mismo por medio de una bomba de analgesia controlada (PCA/venoclisis). Una(un) enfermera(o) le mostrará como usar este simple aparato. También puede pedir medicina si siente nauseas.	Todavía tendrá la bomba de analgesia (PCA) pero también podrá pedir pastillas para el dolor si las necesita (Tylenol). Tal vez empiece a tomar hoy el medicamento anti-coagulante para prevenir coágulos en la sangre. Puede pedir un laxante antes de dormir.	Si no ha obrado (hecho del baño) hasta ahora, le darán un laxante (purgante). La venoclisis (Bomba de analgesia controlada/PCA) se descontinuará pero puede tomar pastillas para el dolor o una inyección si es necesario. Continuará tomando el anticoagulante. Si lo necesita, le darán un laxante suave.	Puede pedir pastillas para el dolor si las necesita. Continuará el protocolo de los anticoagulantes. Si lo necesita, le darán un laxante suave. / Igual que ayer.
Tratamientos	Le pedirán que se talle (cepille) el muslo de la pierna con una solución (ex. Betadina) la noche antes de la operación. No podrá tomar o comer nada o fumar desde la medianoche antes de la operación. Si ha estado tomando aspirina, ibuprofeno u otras medicinas similares, se le pedirá que no las tome por varios días antes de la operación.	Después de la operación, tendrá una almohada de abducción, una almohada regular o algún otro aparato entre las piernas para prevenir la dislocación de la cadera. Se le ayudará a voltearse y a toser fuerte cada dos (2) horas. También se le recordará que use el espirómetro incentivo cada dos (2) horas.	El cuidado de hoy será igual al de ayer. Si no siente nauseas, podrá tomar líquidos hoy. Se le continuará el suero intravenoso para darle fluidos y prevenir que se deshidrate. El tubito de drenaje en la cadera se vaciará y se medirá el líquido cada ocho (8) horas.	Le cambiarán los bendajes de la cadera y el doctor le descontinuará el tubito de drenaje. Necesitará continuar observando las precauciones para la cadera y usando las medias elásticas. Podrá comer lo que desee a menos que esté tomando alimentos especiales (dieta especial).	La(el) enfermera(o) o el técnico le cambiará los bendajes o le limpiará la incisión varias veces al día. Puede comer lo que desee al menos que esté tomando una dieta especial. / Igual que ayer.

Continuada

Guía Para el Paciente: Remplazo Total de la Cadera *Continuada*

Aspecto de Cuidado (Cont.)	Fecha _____ Pre-admisión/ Pre-operativo	Fecha _____ Día 1	Fecha _____ Día 2	Fecha _____ Día 3	Fecha _____ Día 4	Fecha _____ Día 5–6
Tratamientos (Cont.)	Inmediatamente después de la operación se le aplicará un suero intravenoso. Es posible que el doctor ordene una sonda de Foley que usted usará solo durante la operación.	Una persona anotará cuantos líquidos ha tomado y cuanto ha orinado. Le pondrán medias elásticas y aparatos de compresión (SCD/compresión en secuencia) en los dos muslos de las piernas para prevenir cuajarones. Estos aparatos son un poco ruidosos y se sienten muy calientitos. Las(os) enfermeras(os) le ayudarán a mover la pierna opuesta y los brazos para prevenir que se hagan tiesos (duros) o se sientan tensos. Si no puede orinar, le pondrán una sonda para vaciar la vejiga. No podrá comer o tomar nada hasta que despierte por completo, luego le podrán dar líquidos.		El suero intravenoso se le decontinuará hoy.		

Movilidad/Auto Cuidado	No se Aplica.	Se quedará en cama hoy en una posición reclinada. Si necesita obrar (ir al baño), usará un cómodo/bacín pequeño especial para que el movimiento en la cama sea más confortable. Tendrá en la cama un marco y un trapecio para ayudarse a mover por sí mismo. Necesitará hacer los ejercicios para las piernas que le demonstraron.	Hoy lo ayudarán a sentarse al lado de la cama. Después le ayudarán a moverse de la cama a la silla. Elevará la pierna operada/afectada mientras esté fuera de la cama. Se repasarán con usted las precauciones de la cadera, tales como el no cruzar las piernas o pies y el evitar doblarse hacia el frente.	Podrá sentarse hoy (con ayuda) en una silla varias veces al día. Hoy irá al departamento de fisioterapia varias veces al día para empezar ejercicios relacionados con la forma de andar y para caminar con el andador. Deberá usar un sanitario/letrina al lado de la cama o un sanitario con el asiento elevado.	Podrá caminar en su cuarto usando un andador y poniendo un poco de peso en la pierna operada (el técnico de fisioterapia le mostrará cuanto peso poner). Hoy irá al departamento de fisioterapia dos veces para continuar el entrenamiento usando el andador.	Igual que ayer.
Plan al Darle de Alta	No se Aplica.	El(la) trabajor(a) social y la(el) enfermera(o) le hablarán acerca del cuidado en casa antes de ser dado de alta. Dependiendo de su condición y de la situación en su casa, podrá regresar a casa o ir a un centro de rehabilitación/ unidad por cuatro a seis (4-6) semanas.	El(la) trabajor(a) social y la(el) enfermera(o) quienes trabajan con el doctor discutirán los planes para darle de alta. Ellos harán los arreglos para trasladarlo a casa o a un centro de rehabilitación.	Si se le da de alta para regresar a casa, una enfermera y un técnico de fisioterapia le visitarán varias veces por semana. Dependiendo de su situación, usted deberá hacer cita para ir a una consulta externa con un técnico de fisoterapia.	Se le hará una cita para que regrese a ver al doctor. Las(os) enfermeras(os) del hospital se comunicarán con las personas que lo atenderán después de ser dado de alta para repasar con ellos el plan de cuidado.

Guía Para el Paciente: Insuficiencia Renal Aguda: Diálisis Peritoneal

NOTA: Esta guía es solo para el cuidado general. Su cuidado será específico de acuerdo con sus necesidades.

Aspecto de Cuidado	Fecha_____ Día 1	Fecha_____ Día 2	Fecha_____ Día 3	Fecha_____ Día 4	Fecha_____ Día 5
Evaluación	El doctor y la(el) enfermera(o) le harán un examen físico.	El doctor y la(el) enfermera(o) le harán un examen físico.	Igual que ayer.	Igual al día 1.	Igual al día 1.
	La(el) enfermera(o) le hará un examen físico breve al inicio de cada turno.	La(el) enfermera(o) le hará un examen físico breve al inicio de cada turno.			
	Los signos vitales (temperatura, pulso, respiración y la presión de sangre) se le tomarán cada cuatro (4) horas y con más frecuencia mientras reciba el tratamiento de diálisis.	Se le tomarán los signos vitales cada cuatro (4) horas.			
	Se le tomarán los signos neurológicos cada cuatro (4) horas. Esto quiere decir que le:	Los signos neurológi-cos se le tomarán cada cuatro (4) horas.			
	• Pediremos que mueva los brazos y las piernas para ver cuanta fuerza tienen	Le revisaremos con frecuencia para asegurar que no tenga problemas con el diálisis tales como tener el catéter doblado/torcido, o si los bendajes estan mojados.			
		El doctor le ajustará los medicamentos para asegurar que reciba la dósis más adecuada.			

Enseñanza (Instrucción)				
• Apuntaremos una luz en sus ojos para ver como reaccionan • Haremos varias preguntas Le revisaremos con frecuencia para asegurarnos que no tenga problemas con el diálisis tales como sentirse incómodo, tener el catéter doblado/torcido, o si los bendajes están mojados. El doctor le ajustará los medicamentos para asegurar que reciba la dósis más adecuada. Se le preparará a usted y a su familia sobre los procedimientos del diálisis. Se le informará: • Porqué se está haciendo • Como se insertará el catéter peritoneal (abdominal) • Cómo y cuándo se hará el diálisis • Quién lo hará	Las(os) enfermeras(os) le darán información acerca de su diagnóstico, del diálisis y del plan de tratamiento.	Recibirá información acerca de su dieta (alimentos), descanso, y ejercicio. Se le dará información acerca de los medicamentos que necesitará al ser dado de alta. Se le dirá: • El nombre de las medicinas • Cómo y cuándo tomarlas • Para qué son	Repasarán con usted la dieta (los alimentos) y los medicamentos. Los empleados le adiestrarán (darán instrucciones) a usted y a su familia como hacer el diálisis peritoneal en la casa. Si es necesario: • Como hacer el procedimiento	Repasaremos toda la información que necesitará antes de darle de alta.

Continuada

Guía Para el Paciente: Insuficiencia Renal Aguda: Diálisis Peritoneal Continuada

Aspecto de Cuidado (Cont.)	Fecha_____ Día 1	Fecha_____ Día 2	Fecha_____ Día 3	Fecha_____ Día 4	Fecha_____ Día 5
Enseñanza (Instrucción) (Cont.)	• Lo que debe hacer durante el diálisis • Como se siente el diálisis Le diremos como planeamos su cuidado y le pediremos que nos diga qué es lo que podemos hacer para que se sienta mejor. Se le dará información acerca de su diagnóstico.		• Las reacciones adversas que tienen y qué se debe hacer si ocurren.	• Qué hacer y a quién llamar en caso de problemas • Como limpiar el equipo/aparato • Como prevenir infecciones Recibirá un folleto explicando la dieta (los alimentos), medicamentos, ejercicios, actividades y descanso.	
Consultas	El doctor le puede pedir a otros doctores que le visiten a usted. Por ejemplo, al doctor que se especializa en enfermedades del riñón (nefrólogo).	La dietista le visitará para discutir la dieta (alimentos). Nuestro(a), trabajador(a), social le ayudara a entender el seguro médico, los problemas económicos y le puede ayudar a conseguir cuidado en casa.	Igual que ayer.	Ninguna.	Ninguna.
Pruebas de Laboratorio	Se le tomarán muestras de sangre de una vena del brazo al ingresar (ser admitido) al hospital y después de cada procedimiento de diálisis.	Le tomarán muestras de sangre de una vena en el brazo.	Le tomarán muestras de sangre de una vena en el brazo.	Le tomarán muestras de sangre de una vena del brazo. El líquido del catéter en el abdomen se examinará para ver si hay infección.	Le tomarán muestras de sangre de una vena del brazo.

Otros Exámenes	Una muestra de la orina (si es necesario) se mandará al laboratorio para notar si hay infección. El líquido del catéter en su abdomen se examinará para ver si hay infección. Le tomarán rayos-x del pecho y de los riñones. Le tomarán un rayos-x especial llamado CT scan o MRI (resonancia magnética). Le harán un electrocardiograma. Ninguna de estas pruebas le causará molestias.	No se le harán pruebas hoy.	No se le harán pruebas hoy.	Ninguno.	Ninguno.
Medicamentos	Le darán vitaminas con hierro. El doctor ordenará otras medicinas y le diremos que son y cuando debe de tomarlas.	Igual que ayer.	Igual que el día 1.	Los mismos del día 1.	Los mismos del día 1.

Continuada

Guía Para el Paciente: Insuficiencia Renal Aguda: Diálisis Peritoneal *Continuada*

Aspecto de Cuidado (Cont.)	Fecha____ Día 1	Fecha____ Día 2	Fecha____ Día 3	Fecha____ Día 4	Fecha____ Día 5
Tratamientos	Antes del diálisis peritoneal: • Le tomarán los signos vitales • La(el) enfermera(o) le medirá el tamaño del abdomen/cintura • Le pedirán que orine • Le tomarán el peso Durante el diálisis: • Le tomarán los signos vitales • Aseguraremos que el tubo no se doble o que se tape • Si tiene cualquier molestia o problemas al respirar, dígale a las(los) enfermeras(os) Después del diálisis: • Le tomarán los signos vitales • Le tomarán muestras de sangre de una vena del brazo • Se le medirá el abdomen	Recibirá el mismo cuidado que ayer; antes, durante y después del diálisis. Continuaremos midiendo la orina y los líquidos que toma (I & O). Las(os) enfermeras(os) le ayudarán a mover la pierna opuesta y los brazos para prevenir que se hagan tiesos o se sientan tensos. Si no puede orinar, le pondrán una sonda para vaciar la vejiga. No podrá tomar o comer nada hasta que despierte por completo, luego le podrán dar líquidos. Le cambiarán un poco la dieta (los alimentos) dependiendo en su reacción al diálisis.	El cuidado de hoy será igual que ayer. Si hoy no siente náuseas, podrá tomar líquidos. Se continuará el suero intravenoso para darle líquidos y prevenir que se deshidrate. El tubito de drenaje en la cadera se vaciará y se medirá el líquido cada ocho (8) horas. Su dieta (los alimentos) se ajustará para satisfacer sus necesidades.	Igual al día 1.	Igual al día 1.

Continuada

Se le pondrá en I & O lo que quiere decir que se medirán todos los líquidos que tome y también los alimentos como la gelatina, hielo picado y nieve que se consideran líquidos a temperatura ambiente. Se medirá la cantidad que orine cada vez que usa el sanitario/hace del baño.

Dieta (Alimentos):

La dietista discutirá con usted la dieta y le ayudará a seleccionar alimentos bajos en sal y potasio y que tengan la cantidad adecuada de proteina.

Le limitarán la cantidad de líquidos que puede tomar. Los empleados le ayudarán a seleccionar cuando y que podrá tomar.

Una aguja intravenosa se le colocará en una vena del brazo.

Guía Para el Paciente: Insuficiencia Renal Aguda: Diálisis Peritoneal *Continuada*

Aspecto de Cuidado (Cont.)	Fecha_____ Día 1	Fecha_____ Día 2	Fecha_____ Día 3	Fecha_____ Día 4	Fecha_____ Día 5
Movilidad/Auto Cuidado	Puede levantarse para ir al baño/sanitario.	Puede sentarse en una silla el tiempo que pueda y cuanto se sienta cómodo.	Puede levantarse y caminar en los pasillos, si quiere.	Igual al día 3.	Igual al día 3.
Plan al Darle de Alta	Los empleados hablarán con usted acerca del seguro de hospital y de otros problemas económicos.	Los empleados le ayudarán a usted y a su familia a hacer arreglos para lo que necesite al ser dado de alta.	Igual que ayer.	Continuaremos ayudándole a usted y a su familia a identificar cualquier cambio que sea necesario.	Igual al día 3.

Nota

Guía Para el Paciente: Histerectomía Abdominal (Total)

NOTA: Esta guía es solo para el cuidado general. Su cuidado será específico de acuerdo con sus necesidades.

Aspecto de Cuidado	Fecha____ Pre-admisión/ Pre-operativo	Fecha____ Día 1	Fecha____ Día 2	Fecha____ Día 3
Evaluación	Antes de la operación, un(a) enfermero(a) en el quirófano repasará el procedimiento con usted. Le harán un examen físico breve para asegurarse que todo está bien. El(la) enfermero(a) le hará preguntas y le tomará la temperatura, respiración, pulso y presión de sangre. También le pedirán que firme una forma dando permiso para la operación.	Después de la operación, despertará en el cuarto de recuperación (ahora se le llama unidad de post-anestesia o PACU). Las(os) enfermeras(os) en el PACU le tomarán los signos vitales cada 15 minutos al principio de la estancia. Se le despertará y se le revisará con mucha frecuencia. Cuando se despierte por completo, se le transladará a un piso del hospital. Ahí podrá tomar medicina para el dolor y se le continuará revisando cuidadosamente cada 30 a 60 minutos.	Una(un) enfermera(o) le tomará los signos vitales, revisará los bendajes abdominales, y escuchará los sonidos del pecho y de los intestinos al menos cada ocho (8) horas. También se anotará la cantidad de líquidos que toma o que recibe por la intravenosa. Se medirá la cantidad que orina hasta que pueda orinar sin tener dificultad. Le revisarán con frecuencia la toalla sanitaria (para el perineo) para ver cuánto sangra.	Los empleados de enfermería le continuarán examinado el abdomen, el pecho, y le tomarán los signos vitales. También le pedirán que les diga a los empleados cuando haya obrado (hecho del baño).
Enseñanza (Instrucción)	El doctor y los empleados en la oficina le darán instrucciones acera de lo que es una histerectomía y lo que se espera después de la operación.	Le recordarán que respire profundo y que tosa fuerte cuando menos cada dos (2) horas.	Se le adiestrará (darán instrucciones) en métodos para aligerar el dolor tales como relajar los músculos y como formar imágines visuales. Estos métodos no	La(el) enfermera(o) repasará con usted la información que necesitará antes de darle de alta. Debe hacer preguntas si tiene dudas.

	También discutirán lo que ocurrirá después de la operación, tal como el manejo del dolor, cuidado de la incisión (herida), intravenosas y la sonda de Foley. Esta guía para el paciente se deberá repasar con usted y con su familia.	También necesitará usar el espirómetro incentivo cada dos (2) horas y alguien le mostrará como usarlo. Reporte a la(el) enfermera(o) o al asistente cualquier sensación o sangrado fuera de lo común. Por favor haga preguntas se tiene alguna duda.	remplazarán la medicina para el dolor, pero es posible que rebajen la cantidad de medicina que necesite. La(el) enfermera(o) empezará a repasar las instrucciones acerca del cuidado de la incisión, manejo del dolor, actividad, cambios físicos, y medicamentos que tomará cuando regrese a casa.	
Consultas	Ninguna.	Ninguna.	Ninguna.	Ninguna.
Pruebas de Laboratorio	Tendrá que ir al laboratorio varios días antes de la operación para que le tomen muestras de sangre para notar si tiene sangre "baja" (anemia) y si desangra facilmente. También se le pedirá una muestra de la orina.	Un técnico en el laboratorio le tomará muestras de sangre esta tarde o temprano en la mañana para notar si tiene anemia.	Ninguna.	Ninguna.
Otros Examenes	Le tomarán rayos-x del pecho y un electrocardiograma (prueba del corazón) si es mayor de 40 años o si tiene problemas cardiacos.	Ninguno.	Ninguno.	Ninguno.

Continuada

Guía Para el Paciente: Histerectomía Abdominal (Total) Continuada

Aspecto de Cuidado (Cont.)	Fecha_____ Pre-admisión/ Pre-operativo	Fecha_____ Día 1	Fecha_____ Día 2	Fecha_____ Día 3
Medicamentos	Antes de la operación le pondrán una intravenosa para administrarle fluidos, darle medicamentos como los antibióticos y para darle medicina que lo hará sentir adormecido antes de recibir la anestesia. También recibirá muchas medicinas para el corazón. Algunas en forma de pastilla, otras por vía intravenosa y otras que se deben aplicar a la piel.	Después de la operación, el doctor ordenará medicamento para el dolor el cual le aplicarán con inyección o por vía intravenosa por medio de la bomba controlada por el paciente (venoclisis/PCA). Una(un) enfermera(o) le mostrará cómo usar este aparato para que pueda darse, a si mismo, el medicamento para el dolor cuando lo necesite. Es posible que reciba más antibióticos por la vía intravenosa y que tome medicina para náuseas si esta es una molestia.	Si tiene una bomba (PCA) para administrarse medicina para el dolor, es posible que la descontinuen hoy. Puede tomar medicina para el dolor en forma de pastillas/pildoras.	Si no ha obrado (hecho del baño), es probable que le den un supositorio o una enema (lavativa) para ayudarle a obrar.
Tratamientos	El doctor o los empleados en la oficina deben hablar con usted sobre las dudas que tenga acerca de la operación. Le dirán que no tome líquidos, coma alimentos, o fume desde la medianoche (12 de la noche) antes de la operación.	Las(os) enfermeras(os) le darán cuidado del perineo (limpiarle el area) al menos cada ocho (8) horas. Si los bendajes en el abdomen (vientre) se mojan o se aflojan, las(os) enfermeras(os) le pondrán un bendaje sobre el otro para proteger la herida.	Le ayudarán con el aseo del perineo si lo necesita. Deberá cambiar de posición, respirar hondo, y usar el espirómetro. Le permitirán tomar líquidos claros (agua, jugo de manzana, y caldo). Para la cena puede tomar cualquier líquido que desee.	El doctor le cambiará o le quitara hoy los bendajes. Podrá comer o tomar cualquier cosa que desee.

	Se le empezará una vía intravenosa antes de la operación y le pondrán una sonda de Foley para vaciar la vejiga. Después de la operación, le permitirán tomar pedacitos de hielo o traguitos de agua. De otra manera, no podrá comer o tomar líquidos ya que pueden causarle náuseas o mucho malestar.	La bolsa de orina se debe vaciar cada ocho (8) horas y la cantidad se medirá y se anotará en el archivo. Alguien le ayudará a cambiar de posición, a respirar hondo y a toser fuerte cada dos (2) horas. Deberá usar el inspirometro también.	Si pasa gas o si se escuchan sonidos en los intestinos, le permitirán que tome alimentos. Cuando coma y tome bebidas sin tener problemas, le descontinuarán la intravenosa. También le quitarán el catéter de Foley y la revisarán para asegurarse que puede orinar (pasar agua) sin problemas.	
Movilidad/Auto Cuidado	Ninguno.	Si la operación se hizo temprano en la mañana, le ayudarán a sentarse en una silla por la tarde. Le mostrarán cómo hacer ejercicios para las piernas, incluyendo el de punta-talón para prevenir formación de cuajarones. Llevará medias elásticas también para prevenir formación de cuajarones.	Podrá caminar en su cuarto e ir al baño hoy. Si necesita ayuda o se siente mareada, llámele a las(os) enfermeras(os). El doctor le permitirá que se bañe, pero no se deben mojar los bendajes.	Deberá caminar en el cuarto o en el pasillo. Este movimiento le ayudará a disminuir los dolores causados por el "gas." El doctor le permitirá bañarse, pero necesitará mantener seca la incisión (herida).
Plan al Darle de Alta	Ninguno.	Ninguno.	Un(una) trabajador(a) social u otra persona coordinará su salida del hospital y le hablará acerca de necesidades especiales o apoyo que necesite en casa.	El doctor le dará una receta para medicina para el dolor. También le harán una cita para que le quiten las puntadas o las grapas.

Appendix

D

Abbreviations Used in Clinical Pathways

▼ ▼ ▼

ABGs arterial blood gases
ACE angiotensin-converting enzyme
ADA American Diabetic Association
ad lib as tolerated
ADLs activities of daily living
AM morning
amt amount
APTT activated partial thromboplastin time
ASA aspirin

BID twice a day
bicarb bicarbonate
BM bowel movement
BP blood pressure
BRPs bathroom privileges
BSC bedside commode
BSE breast self-exam
BUN blood urea nitrogen

cap capillary
cath catheter
CBC complete blood count
CCU coronary care unit
C & S culture and sensitivity
C-spine cervical spine
CHF congestive heart failure
coag studies coagulation studies
CPK creatine phosphokinase
CPM continuous passive motion
Cr creatinine
CSF cerebrospinal fluid
CT scan computed tomography scan
CVP central venous pressure

5%D/W 5% dextrose in water
5%D/$\frac{1}{2}$NS 5% dextrose in half normal saline
DAT diet as tolerated
D/C discontinue
DB & C deep breathe and cough
DI diabetes insipidus
diff differential
DM diabetes mellitus
DOS day of surgery
DVT deep vein thrombosis

ECF extended care facility
ECG electrocardiogram
EEG electroencephalogram
ELOS expected length of stay
ESR erythrocyte sedimentation rate

FBS fasting blood sugar
F & E fluid and electrolyte
FSBS finger stick blood sugar

g gauge
GM gram

h hour/hours
H$_2$O water
Hct hematocrit
Hgb hemoglobin
HHNC hyperglycemic hyperosmolar nonketotic coma
HOB head of bed

I & O intake and output
ICD-9 international diagnostic code, 9th ed.
ICP intracranial pressure
ICU intensive care unit
INR(PT) international normalized ratio (prothrombin time)
IgE immunoglobulin E
IM intramuscular/-ly
IV intravenous/-ly
IVPB IV piggyback

JP Jackson-Pratt

K$^+$ potassium
KCl potassium chloride
kg kilogram/kilograms
KUB kidneys, ureters, bladder
KVO keep vein open

L liter
lab laboratory
lat lateral
LDH lactic dehydrogenase
LE lower extremity
LOC level of consciousness
LTC long-term care
lytes electrolytes

MD medical doctor/physician
MDI metered dose inhaler
meds medications
Mg^{+2} magnesium
MI myocardial infarction
mL milliliter
min minutes
MRI magnetic resonance imaging
MUGA scan multiunit gated acquisition scan

N/A not applicable
Na$^+$ sodium
NC nasal cannula
neuro neurologic
NGT nasogastric tube
NH nursing home

357

NPO nothing by mouth
NS normal saline
NV neurovascular

O$_2$ oxygen
OB occult blood
OOB out of bed
OR operating room
OT occupational therapy/ therapist

PA posterior/anterior
PACU post-anesthesia care unit
PCA patient-controlled analgesia
PD peritoneal dialysis
PE pulmonary embolus
PM evening
PO by mouth, orally
POD post-operative day
post-op post-operative/-ly
pre-op pre-operative/-ly
PRN as necessary
PT physical therapy/therapist
PTA prior to admission
pulse ox pulse oximetry
PVCs premature ventricular contractions
PWB partial weight-bearing

q every
q h every hour
q 2 h every 2 hours
q 4 h every 4 hours
q 6 h every 6 hours
q 8 h every 8 hours
QD every day
QID four times a day

QOD every other day
quad quadriceps

rehab rehabilitation
ROM range of motion
RUQ right upper quadrant
SaO$_2$ oxygen saturation
SCDs sequential compression devices
SIADH syndrome of inappropriate antidiuretic hormone
SLP speech/language pathologist
SMA-6 (6/60) blood chemistry panel, including lytes, BUN, and glucose
SOB shortness of breath
SP suprapubic
SQ subcutaneous/-ly
S/S signs and symptoms

tab tablet
TCDB turn, cough, deep breathe
temp temperature
TID three times a day
TPN total parenteral nutrition

U/A urinalysis
UE upper extermity

VS vital signs

W/A while awake
WBC white blood cell/count
WNL within normal limits
wt/wts weight/weights

x times

Index

Note: Page numbers in *italics* refer to illustrations; page numbers followed by t refer to tables.